Think Thin, Be Thin

Think Thin, Be Thin

Doris Wild Helmering
and Dianne Hales

BROADWAY BOOKS

NEW YORK

To all who have ever struggled to lose weight

PRINTED IN THE U.S.A.

BROADWAY BOOKS and its logo, a letter B bisected on the diagonal,
are trademarks of Random House, Inc.

Visit our website at www.broadwaybooks.com

First edition published 2005

Book design by Chris Welch

Library of Congress Cataloging-in-Publication Data

Helmering, Doris Wild, 1942–
Think thin, be thin : 101 psychological ways to lose weight / Doris
Helmering and Dianne Hales.— 1st ed.
      p.   cm.
ISBN 0-7679-1696-4
I. Weight loss—Psychological aspects.   I. Hales, Dianne R.,
1950–   II. Title.
RM222.2.H363   2005
613.2'5—dc22   2004058511

Contents

Acknowledgments

Bringing a book to print requires the contributions of many people. We would like to thank Joy Harris, our agent, who was immediately enthusiastic about the idea for this book and who has supported us throughout its creation. Thanks to Jennifer Josephy and Allyson Giard, our editors at Broadway Books, who played an invaluable role in shaping *Think Thin, Be Thin.*

We send special thanks to Pat Gregory at St. Louis University, who allowed herself to be leaned on for research; Judy Cassidy and Roger McWilliams for lending fresh eyes to the material; and special thanks, as always, to Michaeleen Cradock for holding down the fort at the office when Doris was off writing. Gold stars to April Winkelmann, Kate Drewry, Jo Oberreither, Catherine Von Hatten, and Jan Thomas, who all contributed to the process.

A very special thanks to Dr. Robert E. Hales and Dr. Ray Helmering, the two loves of our lives, who as always offered support and encouragement. Love and hugs to Julia Hales and Anna-Mary Helmering and our loving parents. And many more thanks to cheerleaders Layne, Paul,

Sheri, and John Helmering; Korey Hart; Sharon Endejan; Mary Sue Wofford; Mary Jane Lamping; and Martha Scharff, who all gave encouragement and support.

Introduction

Never before have so many had so much to lose. For the first time in history, more than half of the people on the planet are overweight. Obesity, as headlines blare and health experts warn, is the major preventable health threat of the twenty-first century. In the United States alone, obesity annually leads to 300,000 premature deaths and $90 billion in medical costs.

Ironically, as average weights have increased, the quest for thinness has become an obsession. Every year tens of millions of people—15 to 35 percent of Americans, by various estimates—go on diets to lose weight. No matter how much they lose, 90 to 95 percent regain not only the weight they lost but additional pounds. Why?

Our contention, based on decades of scientific research and clinical experience, is that most diets and fitness programs aim at the wrong target: the belly, not the brain. Although they can and do work for a while, these approaches focus on the symptom of weight gain rather than its underlying cause. Diets change what you eat. Exercise changes body composition, stamina, and strength. But changing the brain is the ultimate key to weight loss and control.

Think Thin, Be Thin is the first book to target the neuro-landscape of your brain—the way you think and feel about eating. Unlike diets or weight-loss programs, this book engages the most powerful of tools—the human brain. As you read the information and practice the mental and sensory exercises in *Think Thin, Be Thin*, your brain, which contains hundreds of billions of nerve cells, will develop new neural pathways. As a result, the way you think about food will change, the way you feel about your body will change, and your eating behaviors will change. And you will lose weight.

Are you already on a diet? Have you joined a health club or signed up for a commercial weight-loss program? Don't quit. *Think Thin, Be Thin* complements rather than competes with any diet or fitness plan. As a diet companion, *Think Thin, Be Thin* will put you on track, keep you on track, or help you get back on track. You will eat less, not just because you are following a specific diet, but because you will stop wanting extra food.

Putting Psychology to Work for You

As researchers have demonstrated, hunger has less influence on how much people eat than their attitudes toward food. Changing these attitudes is crucial to changing your eating habits. This is exactly what *Think Thin, Be Thin* does. This book, like its title, may seem simple, but the science behind it is anything but. Every aspect is rooted in rigorously tested, well-established psychological approaches, including:

• **Cognitive-behavior therapy** (CBT), proven the most effective therapy for change and problem solving, emphasizes making changes in the way you think and the way you behave. The premise of CBT is that your thoughts and behaviors—including those related to eating—can be modified in ways that lead to permanent change.

• **Neurolinguistic programming** (NLP), a collection of tools for analyzing how you communicate and organize, filter, and edit information, uses conscious changes in language to create new thinking patterns, which can lead to new eating habits.

• **Compliance theory,** which reveals hidden influences on behavior, helps you recognize and make use of the laws of influence to shed excess pounds.

• **Gestalt therapy** focuses on self-understanding and taking personal responsibility for your behavior, including weight loss and maintenance.

• **Transactional analysis** explores healthy and unhealthy dialogues and interactions that may thwart your efforts to lose weight.

• **Positive psychology,** a relatively new scientific field that studies optimal functioning, helps you develop the strengths that will allow you to control your weight.

• **Naikan and Conscious Living.** These "quiet" therapies, based on Buddhism, redirect the mind away from difficulties and negative feelings toward more productive thoughts and behavior—and a lower weight.

Putting This Book to Work for You

How do we know that the material in *Think Thin, Be Thin* will help you get control of your weight? We've seen it happen when people enter therapy, either individually or in groups, in order to lose weight. Slowly, steadily, sensibly, they lose excess pounds and keep them off.

What is the secret of their success? By applying many and varied psychological strategies—the same ones you'll find in *Think Thin, Be Thin*—they consciously and unconsciously alter their brains. They change the way they think about food. They replace poor eating habits with better ones. They develop alternative ways of coping with stress and stop emotional eating. Even if they have a slow metabolism, even if they were heavy as children, even if all their family members are obese, they take control of their weight—permanently.

The same can happen to you as you read this book. Within these 101 strategies are an additional 550 tips, all crafted to help you reprogram your brain and reach your weight-loss goal. They include such highly effective psychological techniques as meditation, journaling, visualization, and self-hypnosis. Some take the form of suggestions based on the latest scientific findings on weight management. Others consist of mental exercises, such as affirmations, metaphors, quizzes, and parables. With so many weight-loss strategies and solutions in these pages, you are sure to find some that will work for you.

Think back to when you learned to drive: You were conscious of every step—inserting the key in the ignition, putting the car in gear, releasing the emergency brake. But starting the car soon became automatic. The reason? You unconsciously changed the neural pathways of your brain. This same process will happen to you as you read and practice the exercises in *Think Thin, Be Thin.*

Don't expect an immediate transformation or a quick drop in weight. However, as you read and complete some of the assignments, you will learn to peer inside your brain. You will become conscious of the words, phrases, and messages you use to talk to yourself. You will step back from yourself and "see," perhaps for the first time, the ways in which you use food. You will become aware of the thoughts you think about eating at the very moment you're thinking them. And you will learn to manipulate and replace them with healthier thoughts.

You can read *Think Thin, Be Thin* in tiny bites or big chunks. We urge you to take the time to read the first fifteen entries and then "work" your way through the book. As you do, exposure to so many pieces of information will continue to create new neural pathways and connections. Your brain will take control of your eating behavior. You will no longer eat mindlessly. You will go on fewer food binges. You will make different food choices. You will exercise more. And you will lose weight.

1

101 Ways to Change

One of the truisms of psychology is that a problem never has just one cause, but rather stems from many causes. Just as there is no single cause for a problem, there is no one solution. For most problems, there are many solutions that can and do work.

This is especially true for weight.

Because each individual is different, a diet, a therapeutic technique, a concept, a suggestion, or an exercise program that helps one person lose weight may be unappealing or ineffective with another. However, when offered many weight-loss strategies and solutions, almost everyone will find one, or several, that work.

The basic premise of *Think Thin, Be Thin* comes from the "mere exposure effect," the well-documented principle that the more you see, hear, or read a message, the more positively you view it. The logos for Coca-Cola and Nike appear the world over because their manufacturers realize that mere exposure elicits a positive response to a brand or product. However, at some point, we stop paying attention to the same message presented over and over in the same fashion. We crave novelty and variety. That's why the debut of new commercials on Super Bowl Sunday draws almost as many viewers as the action on the field.

This book repeatedly exposes you to the simple concept that you can control your weight. Because no one strategy will work for every reader, we offer 101 fresh and varied weight-loss alternatives. Although you may not be aware of what's happening, mere exposure to these options will open your mind to the possibility that you can change the way you deal with food. And something in these pages—an insight, a technique, or a new approach— is sure to inspire you. When you make just one small change, you open the door to more changes.

This is not wishful thinking. Compliance experts, who study how people are influenced, know that once a person believes that change is possible, change occurs. With each change, you will come to see yourself as someone who can take charge of your weight. Through this process of self-indoctrination, you will develop a new inner responsibility for your body that will take on a momentum of its own.

The first step we recommend doesn't even involve food. Buy a "Think Thin, Be Thin" notebook, and write the following sentence on the first page:

"I, _____, will continue to read *Think Thin, Be Thin* and put some of the suggestions to work for me."

If you prefer, open a new "Think Thin, Be Thin" file on your computer, type the sentence, and print it out. Either way, sign your name and record the date. Doing so creates a subtle, subconscious pressure to follow through on your agreement. With one small commitment, you psychologically prime yourself to make other commitments that will lead to a thinner, healthier you.

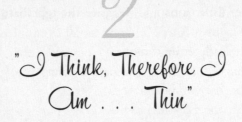

"I Think, Therefore I Am . . . Thin"

Diet experts emphasize that if you want a healthier, trimmer body, you should eat less and exercise more. They're right. But how do you get yourself to eat less and exercise more?

The answer lies in your brain. Your thoughts determine how you feel. Your thoughts determine how you behave. Your thoughts determine what you eat and whether you work out.

The discovery that thoughts create feelings and drive behavior—one of the most important psychological breakthroughs of the last fifty years—is the foundation of all cognitive and behavioral therapy approaches. Although these methods were developed separately, they all place heavy emphasis on setting goals (defining what you intend to accomplish) and changing the way you think about or interpret a situation.

Every day, according to neuroscientists, each of us thinks about sixty thousand thoughts as we plan, evaluate, judge, interpret, and remember. Some of our thoughts are as precise and logical as mathematical equations. Others are misleading or inappropriate. These inaccurate or self-defeating thoughts are the targets of cognitive-behavior therapy (CBT), which helps individuals free themselves from the distortions and negative thought patterns that shape their lives.

We do not contend that you can think yourself thin. But we know that changes in your thoughts can shape the behaviors that will enable you to change and lose weight. *Think Thin, Be Thin* focuses on changing your thinking about weight, food, and health, which will lead directly to a change in your behavior.

If you think that you can shed excess pounds, if you think that you can control what you put in your mouth, if you think that there is a form of exercise that you could enjoy, if you think that you can get back on your diet, then you are on your way to reaching your weight-loss goals. Throughout this book we will show you how to change and adjust the ways you think so you can change and adjust the ways you behave—and lose weight.

3

Where Are You?

How will you change as you read this book? Stage by stage. In more than twenty years of research on motivational readiness for change, behavioral scientists have identified five distinct stages that people move through as they go from clueless, to conscious, to committed to transforming their lives.

If you are still in the *precontemplation* stage, something is gnawing at you, but you aren't sure why you feel such unrest. You don't think of yourself as having a weight problem, even though others may. If you can't fit into some of your clothes, you blame the cleaners. Or you look around and think, "I'm no bigger than anyone else in the office." Unconsciously you may feel helpless to do anything about your weight. So you deny or dismiss its importance.

In the *contemplation* stage, you would prefer not to have to change but you can't avoid reality. Your doctor may caution you about your weight or high blood pressure. You wince at the vacation photos of you in a swimsuit. You look in the mirror, try to suck in your stomach, and say, "I've got to do something about my weight." Not tomorrow, you tell yourself, but definitely in the next six months.

In the *preparation* stage, you're gearing up by taking small but necessary steps. You may join a health club, buy athletic shoes, check out several diet books from the library, or call a commercial weight-loss program for information. Maybe you experiment with some minor changes, such as not eating a snack before bed or going to a yoga class with a friend. Internally you are getting accustomed to the idea of change. Maybe you even mark a "D" (for diet) day on your calendar.

In the *action* stage of change, you are deliberately working to lose weight. You no longer snack at your desk. You stick to a specific diet and track calories, carbs, or points. You hop on a treadmill or stationary bike for thirty minutes a day. You remind yourself a thousand times a day that no food could ever taste as good as being thin will feel. Your resolve is strong, and you know you're on your way to a thinner, healthier you.

In the *maintenance* stage, you strengthen, enhance, and extend the changes you've made. Whether or not you have lost all the weight you want, you've made significant progress. As you continue to watch what you eat and to be physically active, you lock in healthy new habits.

Where are you right now? Read each statement and decide which best applies to you.

1. I'm standing in the bookstore *Contemplation* flipping through this book *Stage* because I'd like to lose weight.

2. I bought this book and I'm probably *Preparation* going to try some of the suggestions. *Stage*

3. I have been following a diet for   *Action*
   three weeks and have started   *Stage*
   working out.

4. I have been sticking to a diet and   *Maintenance*
   engaging in regular physical activity   *Stage*
   for at least six months.

Don't expect to progress through these stages just once. Most people "recycle" several times before a change becomes permanent. As you do so, different strategies in this book may prove more useful than others at different times. Cognitive strategies, such as learning about the risks of excess weight, typically work best in the contemplation and preparation stages. Cognitive and behavioral strategies, such as positive self-talk, journaling, keeping a food diary, or putting down your fork between bites, are more effective in the action and maintenance stages.

Whether you're moving forward or have temporarily fallen back, remember that change is a journey that happens step by step, meal by meal, day by day, stage by stage.

4

Your Line in the Sand

Stand alone in a room. Draw an imaginary line in front of yourself. The side you're standing on represents your past weight issues. The other side of the line represents the life that is yours to shape and change. Maybe you already crossed this line psychologically when you started to read *Think Thin, Be Thin.* If you have not yet crossed the line, choose a position in relation to the line and note how it feels to be where you are now.

Do you know how far you are from crossing the line? Can you visualize yourself crossing? Then answer the following questions:

• Is something in the way of your crossing? Maybe you can't afford to join a gym or sign up for a commercial weight-loss program. If so, are you ready to look for a no- or low-cost alternative, such as walking in a park every morning? If not, when might you be ready?

• Do you need to do anything before crossing? Maybe you're planning a big party and figure you'd blow your diet preparing the feast. Why not ask a friend or family members to help with the cooking so you're less likely to be tempted?

• Is there any other reason to postpone crossing? Maybe part of you is afraid of trying and failing, especially if that's happened before. Are you afraid of what lies on the other side? For instance, you may worry that others will expect you to take on more responsibilities, such as leading school hikes or volunteering for charity walkathons, if you slim down. Think through how you might handle such requests—or consider the idea that you might even enjoy such outings.

Psychologist Kenneth W. Christian, author of *Your Own Worst Enemy*, developed this exercise for the Maximum Potential Project, which helps people overcome self-limiting behavior. As he and others have found, there is seldom any advantage to deferring change. If you wait until you have more money, more time, or you're comfortable with what the future holds, you may end up waiting forever. So go ahead. Cross the line.

5

Transform Wishes into Goals

If we could wish away weight, none of us would be heavy. Unfortunately, lots of overweight people live in wish mode. You may wish that you didn't have such a big appetite, that you didn't enjoy food so much, or that you had more time to exercise. But you're more likely to slim down if you stop wishing and take concrete steps toward what you want.

In research on performance in students, athletes, and employees, the one characteristic that separates high and low achievers is having clear, specific goals. As you launch your weight-loss program, set goals that are both a reach and reachable. As you progress, add or modify your goals so they continue to inspire rather than overwhelm you.

Here are our suggestions for creating goals worth going for:

• **See it, say it, and write it.** Create an image of your goal. Maybe you see yourself dazzling old friends at a reunion or buttoning the pants that fit just last year. Maybe you visualize yourself smiling as you step on a scale or see your lithe body in a bikini. Describe and define your goal in your mind. Then put it in words, and commit it to paper. Until you write down what you want, it's only a wish.

Set aside a page or section of your notebook to record, amend, modify, refine, expand, and extend your goals—and to check off each one as you reach it.

• **Think in terms of evolution, not revolution.** Revolutionary changes trigger counterrevolutionary rebellion. Although you may want to drop fifteen, twenty-five, fifty pounds or more, aim for losing five. Anticipate the sense of accomplishment you'll feel as you hit each five-pound marker. Each small win can add up to a big boost in motivation. Even if you want to shed more pounds, this difference alone will lower your health risks and boost your self-confidence.

• **Identify your resources.** Do you have what you need—knowledge, skills, time—to succeed? For instance, if you're committing yourself to a daily walk, make sure you have good shoes. Identify a path or track. Decide if you'll go alone or ask a friend to join you. Clear thirty minutes of your day so you'll be sure to hit the trail.

• **Systematically analyze barriers.** Think through, in very concrete and specific terms, what is likely to get in your way. For each obstacle, list solutions. If bad weather is a potential threat, for instance, come up with indoor alternatives. If the break room at work always overflows with goodies, limit the time you spend there, or bring a healthy snack. If seeing other people eat high-calorie foods makes you crave them, eat lunch with a friend who's also watching his or her weight.

• **Set goals that go beyond pounds.** Thinking only in terms of pounds can be both limiting and frustrating. Set goals that focus on changing behavior and make them as specific as possible, for example:

Today's goal: I will take a fifteen-minute walk at lunchtime, and I'll have low-fat milk instead of a milk shake with my lunch.

This week's goal: At least three evenings this week, I'll have fruit for dessert or no dessert at all.

This month's goal: I'm going to get off the bus one stop sooner and walk the rest of the way to and from work. If the weather's bad, I'll walk up one flight before taking the elevator up to my office or apartment. By the end of the month, I'll get off two stops away and walk two or three flights before getting on the elevator.

6

The Miracle of the Affirmation

"Every day in every way, I'm getting better and better."

You may have heard this phrase so often that you dismiss it as a cliché of pop "feel good" psychology. It's not.

In the early 1920s Emile Coúe, a French therapist, developed a technique called conscious autosuggestion, which required repeating this phrase twenty times on awakening and twenty times before retiring. Through the years, researchers around the world have confirmed that repeating a positive statement affects self-perceptions and self-esteem. Frequent repetition of an affirmation, a motivating phrase or sentence, has become a fundamental part of cognitive-behavior therapy.

When you are trying to lose weight, saying an affirmation over and over in your head is one of the fastest ways to restructure your thought patterns, develop new pathways in your brain, and change your mind-set about food.

To affirm your way to a lower weight and a fitter body, try one of the following:

- "I am healthy, work out, and eat carefully."
- "I am physically active and limit what I put in my mouth."
- "I'm on my way to a thinner, healthier, happier me."

If none of these affirmations suits you, make up one of your own. Your affirmation should be positive, use the present tense, and target the change you desire. Write down your affirmation, and be sure to make the phrase as clear and compelling as possible. Then say it to yourself.

How often? You'll need to repeat your affirmation about an hour each day the first week, and then fifteen or twenty minutes each day for a few months for reinforcement. Say your affirmation while doing any simple task— while taking a shower, blow-drying your hair, sitting in traffic, emptying the dishwasher, waiting for the subway, riding an elevator.

Although you aren't conscious of what is happening, your affirmation will create a new pathway of connections in your brain. Within a few days, you'll find that you don't think so often about taking a second helping or skipping your exercise class. As you keep repeating your affirmation, you'll feel a greater desire to eat right and exercise more.

Does it sound too good to be true? Put this technique to the test for the next five days. You have nothing to lose but pounds.

7

Eat Less or Exercise More?

S ome women would rather restrict what they eat than work up a sweat. Others prefer to move their muscles and not worry about what they put in their mouths. Which approach works better? That depends on your goals.

To improve your health and lower your risk of death and disease, exercise has proven more beneficial.

To shed pounds, you have to cut back on how much you eat so you're consuming fewer calories than you expend.

If you increase exercise without decreasing food intake, you will improve fitness, build lean muscle mass, and reduce body fat. But don't expect your scale to register a major change.

If you eat less but don't exercise, you will lose pounds, but about one quarter of the lost weight will come from muscle tissue rather than fat—and you're more likely to regain whatever you lose because, as you lose muscle, your metabolic rate slows down.

It's not a question of either/or but of doing both. According to recent research, a combination of dietary change and a moderate to high level intensity of exercise leads to greater weight loss than either alone.

If you decide to exercise and cut back on calories, how long will it take you to get where you want your weight to be? That depends on how much you do and how many calories you cut. Use the chart below to figure it out.

Countdown
Days to Lose Weight

If you walk (minutes)	If you cut daily calories by	5 lb	10 lb	15 lb	20 lb	25 lb
30	400	27	54	81	108	135
30	800	16	32	48	64	80
45	400	23	46	69	92	115
45	800	14	28	42	56	70
60	400	21	42	63	84	105
60	800	13	26	39	54	65

8

Change to the Language of Change

Every day we unconsciously hypnotize ourselves with the words we use when we talk to ourselves and to others. These messages can paralyze or inspire, mire us down or move us forward. Pay attention both to what you say when you talk or think about weight and to how you say it. Then consciously edit the words in your mind and your mouth.

• **Watch out for weasel words.** Are you "planning" to go on a diet? "Hoping" to lose weight? "Trying" to slim down?

What's wrong with these phrases? They all reveal ambivalence and doubt. When you use linguistic loopholes like "trying" or "hoping," you give yourself permission to settle for whatever happens. Push the delete key in your mind. When you speak of goals, use definitive, unequivocal language. Say, "I will lose weight," not "I would like to lose weight." Cut the flab from the way you talk about weight.

• **Trade tenses.** When thinking or talking about your weight struggles, switch to the past tense. Instead of saying, "I'm too lazy to exercise," tell yourself, "I used to be too lazy to exercise." Instead of "I always blow my diets," switch to "I used to blow my diets." Changing the tense helps you differentiate between what you did in the past and what is possible now. You remind yourself that you have changed, are changing, or at the least are capable of change.

When speaking positively about your body and health, use the present tense, even for behaviors you haven't adapted—yet. Tell yourself: "I am changing the way I live," "I am eating healthfully," "I am losing weight."

• **Switch from "why" to "how."** Instead of using the word "why" to explain your actions, switch to "how." For example, if you ask yourself why you overeat, you might answer, "Things aren't going well in my life," or "I get bored in the evening."

If you ask yourself how you overeat, you might answer, "I take second helpings," "I snack when I watch television," or "I eat all day long at my desk."

The next time you reach for another helping or a snack, thoughts of how you are overeating may surface rather than another excuse for why you're doing so.

• **Not "if" but "when."** People who are struggling to lose weight often sabotage themselves by saying, "if" or "if only." "If I could lose twenty-five pounds." "If only I had more willpower." Such statements reinforce the notion that you're never going to lose weight.

Instead of another "if," say to yourself, "When I lose twenty-five pounds," "When I'm thin," or "When I start working out." This simple switch sets the stage for believing that you will be able to change your lifestyle and lose weight.

• **Just "because."** According to social psychology research, using the word "because" when making a request or seeking agreement can boost your compliance as high as 80 to 90 percent. Even when you talk to yourself, using the word "because" shifts your brain to a deeper level of analysis. For instance, you might tell yourself:

> "I'll eat smaller portions of food *because* I want to lose weight."
> "I'll do some form of exercise each day *because* I want to be strong and flexible."
> "I won't buy sweet rolls *because* I don't want to be tempted."

Now it's your turn. Jot these sentences in your notebook.

I'll _____ because _____.

I'll _____ because _____.

9

Observe Yourself

What if a private investigator watched you for a day? How would such an impartial observer view your eating habits?

This "watcher" might notice that you eat three or four cookies while preparing dinner, that you eat faster than anyone else at the table, and that if there is a cake in the house, you nibble at it until it's gone. An impartial observer also might see that, even though you are dieting, you eat half of your spouse's dessert.

To gain the insights only someone on the sidelines can offer, for the next week become your own impartial observer. Each hour on the hour, preface your thoughts, feelings, and behavior with the words "*I am aware . . .*" For example:

I am aware that I'm eating a bagel with cream cheese.
I am aware of feeling hassled and treating myself to a candy bar.
I am aware of buying a bag of chips from the vending machine because I started dozing off at my desk.
I am aware that I'm choosing between bottled water and another can of soda.

You can use this technique at any stage of a diet. In the beginning, it will help you spot mindless, out-of-control eating. As you progress, observing yourself will reveal behaviors that are slowing your weight loss.

10

Plan to Lose

Ask winners the secret of their success in academics, business, or sports, and they consistently say they start with a plan. If you want to win the weight-loss wars, you have to plan to lose. We suggest not just one master plan, but several:

• **Make a weekly plan.** Every Sunday make a meal plan for the coming week. List the foods you need to buy. Whether you're counting calories, fat grams, carbohydrates, or points, figure out the calculations for each day's meals and snacks. Factor in business lunches, family get-togethers, or dinners out. Post this meal plan on your refrigerator door. Check off each meal and day. If your eating doesn't go exactly according to plan, make adjustments as you plan the next day.

• **Plan for tomorrow.** Before you go to bed, make a healthy to-do list for the next day. Write down in your "Think Thin, Be Thin" notebook what you'll eat and how you'll work in some exercise. Compliance experts know that if people actually put down on paper a list of what they intend to do, they're more likely to follow through.

If you forgot to plan the night before, make up a menu in the morning, and stick to it so you aren't focusing on food later in the day when you're tired and hungry. Too busy to do this in the morning rush? Before every meal, jot down on a Post-it note what you plan to eat. Keep it in sight (or at least in mind) as you prepare your meal at home or order in a restaurant.

• **Plan your indulgences.** List the foods you adore even though you know they aren't great for your diet or health. Rank your five favorites in order of their importance to you. Allow yourself to eat the top two or three but not the others. Plan how often (we suggest no more than once a week) and how much you'll eat of them. To stick to this limit, buy a single-serving bag of chips or the smallest carton of ice cream. Order a half-size portion of your favorite restaurant entrée. This strategy flexes your self-control muscles without triggering what influence experts call the "Romeo and Juliet" effect of increasing your desire for anything you can't have.

11

Who's in Charge?

Do you see yourself as master of your fate, asserting control over your destiny? Or do so many things happen in your life that you just hang on and hope for the best? The answers to these questions reveal two important characteristics that affect your weight: your locus of control (the sense of being in control of your life) and your sense of self-efficacy (the belief in your ability to change and to reach a goal).

Hundreds of studies have compared people who have different perceptions of control. "Internals," who believe that their actions largely determine what happens to them, act more independently, enjoy better health, and are more optimistic about their future. "Externals," who perceive that chance or outside forces determine their fate, find it harder to cope with stress and feel increasingly helpless over time. When it comes to weight, they see themselves as destined to be fat.

Feeling in control goes hand in hand with belief in ability to change. In his research on self-efficacy, psychologist Albert Bandura of Stanford University found that the individuals most likely to reach a goal are those who believe that they can. The stronger their faith in themselves, the more energy and persistence they put into making a change. The opposite is also true, especially for health behaviors. In one study of people who began an exercise program, those with lower self-efficacy were more likely to drop out.

How do you rate on locus of control and self-efficacy? Read the following questions and jot down True or False in your notebook:

1. I am overweight because I eat too much.
2. Weight problems run in my family.
3. Diet pills are my best hope for losing weight.
4. I would keep weight off if I exercised regularly.
5. I wouldn't overeat if I didn't have to cook for my family.
6. Some people are born thin and never have to diet.
7. I lose weight when I eat only diet shakes or prepared foods.
8. I could make time for exercise if I really wanted to.
9. My doctor will make sure I'm at a healthy weight.
10. I'm determined to lose weight, and I know I will.

True answers to numbers 1, 4, 8, and 10 indicate that you take responsibility for and see yourself in control of your weight. True answers to numbers 2, 3, 5, 6, 7, and 9 suggest that you credit or blame others for your weight. The more that you see external forces as in charge, the more difficult you will find it to make changes and lose weight permanently.

Many of the psychological strategies in *Think Thin, Be Thin* can help shift your locus of control and boost your sense of self-efficacy. After reading more of this book and trying some of our recommendations, retake this quiz. Your answers may reflect a new way of thinking about yourself, your weight, and the possibility of change.

12
Try Sensory Representation

What is your learning style?

If you're a visual learner, you learn best by watching, observing, and using your eyes to see information. You are good at seeing colors, remembering faces, playing cards or chess, and doing crossword puzzles. You are technologically and mathematically inclined.

If you are an auditory learner, you best learn and remember information you hear. Because of your fine-tuned ear, you have a good vocabulary, articulate ideas well, and may be adept at languages and music.

What does your sensory learning style have to do with weight loss? A great deal. Psychologists refer to the use of words that allow you to see or hear as "sensory representation." The more often you choose words that are right for you, the more your brain will help you achieve your goal.

Saying "I must exercise," for instance, does not set up an imaginary picture or an auditory prompt in the brain. "I'm going to run on the beach today," on the other hand, creates a sensory representation you can see. If you add, "I'll listen to the sound of the surf," you set up an additional sensory representation you can hear.

This technique can help prevent diet lapses. Before a dinner out, you might say to yourself, "I will order a salad with lemon instead of dressing, poached salmon, steamed asparagus, and an espresso for dessert." To add an auditory prompt, you might hear the waiter ask for your order and hear yourself say, "I'd like the salmon."

Sensory representation works because creating mental pictures triggers electrochemical changes that prime your brain into translating your sensory thoughts into action. Try this simple practice exercise:

- Read the following words: "Think thin, be thin."
- Write them down, and read them several times.
- Say the words out loud.

In a few seconds, you've used visual and auditory cues to reinforce the message of this book.

13
Your Food Diaries

A food diary, like the one in the Appendix, can serve different purposes at different points in your weight-loss program. Often people resist keeping a food log because they don't want to know exactly how much they eat. But if you really want to lose weight, you have to take the mystery out of your food life. An added incentive: In studies of dieters, keeping a diary often helped people lose weight because it forced them to be accountable for their food choices.

• **If you are thinking about or starting a diet.** Use your food diary as a research tool. Without changing your usual routine or judging yourself, in your notebook record when, where, why, and how much you eat. After a week, analyze the data. Look for patterns and problems. Are you skipping breakfast? Do you snack all day long on weekends? Are you consuming more calories than you would have guessed? Where do they come from? The answers can provide valuable information as you launch your weight-loss program.

• **If you're on a diet.** Use your food diary as a periodic reality check that provides a snapshot of your food intake.

For three days (including one weekend day), tally your daily total in calories, carbs, points, or fat grams. Are they higher than your diet allows? Highlight every "diet-right" choice you've made. Circle every diet stumble or no-no. Don't criticize yourself for less-than-perfect compliance. Just use the new information to fine-tune your weight-loss strategies.

• **If you hit a plateau.** Use your food diary to figure out why. For a week, conscientiously record every morsel that you eat—down to each lick of icing or cake batter. If your diary reveals that you're a food sneak thief, catch yourself before you take a bite. Keep Post-it notes around the house, at your desk, and in your purse to remind yourself to write down everything you put in your mouth. Simply knowing you have to do so can discourage you from sneaking a treat.

• **If you overeat.** Use your food diary to overcome what we call "overboard" eating, when you just can't stop stuffing yourself. Each time you overeat, write an O for overboard. If you go overboard three times in a day, you'll have three O's. If you cross over the line five times, put down five O's. Recording overeating will help you become more conscious of just how much you're putting in your mouth. As your awareness grows, you can expect to go overboard far less often.

• **If you'd like support.** Use your food diary to connect with others. If you have a weight-loss buddy, swap food diaries occasionally. Some people post their food logs online or share them with a support group. We've found that, despite their initial embarrassment, people in our weight-loss groups get in the spirit of giving "attaboys" for days of healthy eating and laughing at slips such as breakfasts of tiramisu or carrot cake. As the weeks go by, they also find themselves making healthier food choices.

14

The Foot in the Door

L ook at the list of behavioral changes below, and think through how difficult they would be to implement. Assign each a number from I to IO, indicating degree of difficulty, with IO the most challenging and I the least. Eliminate those that are already part of your weight-loss program.

Choose one change and commit to it. You may want to tackle the toughest first or start with the easiest and work up to harder ones. But whatever you choose, focus on just one change. Add another only after the previous one has become part of your life.

- Replace bad fats (e.g., butter) with good fats (e.g., olive oil).
- Eat one more daily serving of fresh fruits or vegetables.
- Cut your portion size by a third.
- Eliminate second helpings.
- Add one workout to your weekly exercise regimen.
- Eat one fewer restaurant meal a week.
- Replace soda and other "snack drinks" with water.
- Learn to cook a healthy new dish.

- Remove all unhealthy snacks from your cupboards.
- Try a new exercise class or activity.

Write your first change in your "Think Thin, Be Thin" notebook or file. Each day make it one of the top priorities on your to-do list.

By implementing several of these foot-in-the-door suggestions, you pave the way for greater behavioral changes in the future. By writing down your intended change, you're more likely to follow through and make it happen.

15

No More Negatives

If you had a friend who was trying to lose weight, would you call her a fat slob? Would you tell her she's worthless and has no self-control? Would you point out that she probably always will be fat, just like her mother?

Of course not, but chances are you've said those things—or worse—to yourself. The self-talk of people who fail to lose weight is notoriously negative. They tend to have and express a negative view of themselves, a negative interpretation of current experiences, and a negative outlook on the future. What they don't realize is that negative thinking is trapping them in their overweight bodies by programming their brains for failure.

Negative thoughts are self-defeating because they refer only to where you are at a certain moment. If you say to yourself, "I've always been on the heavy side," or "I've never been able to lose much weight," you don't allow any possibility for change. If you keep recycling such thoughts, you'll be just as heavy, if not heavier, a year, two years, three years from now. If you want to lose weight and keep it off, you must eliminate the negative thoughts that keep you stuck. Here's how:

• **Guard against demeaning words and phrases.** When a derogatory statement about yourself forms in your brain, say firmly, "Stop!" or "Delete!" If this is a hard habit to break, wear a rubber band on your wrist and snap it to alert yourself that you are thinking negative, debilitating thoughts.

• **Don't focus on what you can't do.** People in our weight-loss groups often complain that they "can't stand" exercising or going without sweets. The fact is that you can stand almost anything. Remind yourself of your strengths every day. Say to yourself, "I can stand this diet," "I can stand another ten minutes on the treadmill," "I can stand living without *fettucine alfredo.*"

• **Turn negative thoughts into hopeful but realistic statements.** If you hear yourself say, "I can't lose weight," replace the statement with, "Right now I'm not losing weight, but when I decide to do it, I will." Jot down any negative observations you make about your body or weight in your notebook to increase your awareness and give you the chance to prepare a counterattack the next time you hear them.

• **Toss the thought away.** If you keep calling yourself a fatso or berating yourself for not having any willpower, write the thought on paper and shred it, burn it, or crumble and throw it away. This symbolic gesture will remind you to get rid of all the negative thoughts that creep into your head.

• **Give yourself two positives for each negative.** People remember negative comments far more than they remember positive ones. In order to counteract this psychological phenomenon, give yourself two positive strokes or compliments for every putdown. If you find yourself saying, "I'm such a loser," remind yourself that you speak two languages or have a garden that is the envy of the neighborhood.

16

Which Way Is the Best Weigh?

Are you overweight or, as some contend, "under-height"?

The answer isn't always clear because of controversy and confusion over the ideal weights for various heights. Rather than rely on a range of ideal weights for various heights, as they did in the past, medical experts use body mass index (BMI), a ratio between weight and height that correlates with percentage of body fat. (You can check your BMI on the chart in the Appendix.)

A healthy BMI ranges from 18.5 to 24.9. A BMI of 25 or greater defines overweight. If your BMI is between 25 and 29.9, your weight is undermining the quality of your life. You suffer more aches and pains. You find it harder to perform everyday tasks. You run a greater risk of serious, potentially lethal health problems, including high blood pressure, arteriosclerosis, diabetes, gallbladder disease, respiratory disease, arthritis, gout, congestive heart failure, infertility, and urinary incontinence.

A BMI of 30 or greater defines obesity. If your BMI is over 30, you face all these dangers plus one more: dying prematurely. Every year about 400,000 Americans die of weight-related problems. Unless you lower your BMI, you're likely to join them sooner rather than later.

BMI is reliable for most, but not all people. If you're pregnant or nursing, extremely muscular, or elderly, BMI is not a good measure of health risks. As a better option, some experts recommend monitoring body fat, which typically increases with age as lean muscle decreases. Too little muscle means less energy, stamina, and strength. Too much body fat means higher risk of health problems, particularly if you store fat around your midsection.

You can check your body fat in various ways. Hand-held body-fat analyzers, sold at specialty stores or online, give a roughly reliable estimate. Many gyms and health clubs have stand-on body fat monitors. Athletic trainers and health professionals traditionally have used calipers to calculate body fat. Once you find out your body fat percentage, use the chart below to see if your body fat is in the healthy range for your age.

Body Fat Percentages for Women

	Minimum	Maximum
Age 20–29	16	24
Age 30–39	17	25
Age 40–49	19	28
Age 50–59	22	31
Age 60+	22	33

Source: American College of Sports Medicine

17

Waist Not

Pay attention to your waist as well as your weight. Even if your scale shows that you haven't gained a lot of weight, your waist may widen—particularly if you've been under stress. Because of the physiological impact of stress hormones, fat accumulates around your midsection in times of tension and turmoil.

A widening waist, or "apple" shape, is a warning signal. Unlike fat in the thighs or hips, abdominal fat increases the risk of high blood pressure, type 2 diabetes, high cholesterol, and metabolic syndrome (a perilous combination of overweight, high blood pressure, and high levels of cholesterol and blood sugar). To measure your waist circumference, place a tape measure around your bare abdomen just above your hipbone. Be sure that the tape is snug but does not compress your skin. Relax, exhale, and measure.

When is a waist too wide? Various studies have produced different results, but the general guideline is that a waist measuring more than 35 inches in a woman or more than 40 inches in a man signals greater health risks.

Another way of determining your health risk is your waist-to-hip ratio, or WHR. In addition to measuring your waist, measure your hips at the widest part. Divide your hip measurement into your waist measurement. For women, a ratio of 0.80 or less is considered safe; for men, the recommended ratio is 0.90 or less. For both men and women, a 1.0 or higher is considered "at risk," or in the danger zone, for undesirable health consequences such as heart disease and other ailments associated with being overweight.

18

Are You Weight Wise?

What's your weight-loss intelligence quotient? Take the following twelve-point test now, when you finish *Think Thin, Be Thin,* and a few months later.

In your journal write the numbers one to twelve along the margin. Give yourself a checkmark each time you can answer a question with a yes. Otherwise leave the space next to the number blank.

1. I am almost always conscious of what I eat.
2. When I get up in the morning, I plan a time for exercise.
3. If I overindulge at one meal, I don't continue to overeat for the rest of the day.
4. I don't blame my genes or others for my weight problem, because I am responsible for what I put in my mouth.
5. I don't buy or eat sweets, chips, or other snacks on a regular basis.
6. I don't eat fast food more than twice a week.
7. I make sure to eat five servings of fruits and vegetables each day.

8. I have a good idea how many calories, carbohydrates, fat, and protein are in most foods I eat regularly.

9. I weigh myself every week to monitor my weight. If I've gained more than three pounds, I immediately eat less or exercise more.

10. I rarely use food as comfort. Instead I do something else and remind myself that the bad, sad, or mad feeling will pass.

11. I use a number of psychological techniques, such as affirmations, journaling, or meditation, to control my eating.

12. I don't allow myself to sit for more than an hour before I get up and walk, stretch, or bend.

How did you do? If you only had four check marks, that's okay. Keep reading *Think Thin, Be Thin* and using the suggestions. The next time you take this test, you'll have more. Eventually you'll score a perfect twelve.

19

Discover the Joys of Journaling

Putting feelings into words and words onto paper is a powerful tool for behavior change. The process of expressive writing, or journaling, provides an opportunity to reflect, evaluate past, present, and future behavior, and gain insight into your feelings. Writing about your inner life often has a positive effect on both mental and physical health.

A psychological journal can be the secret weapon in your weight-loss program. Unlike a food diary, which tracks what goes into your mouth, a psychological journal explores what's going on in your mind. A psychological journal focuses not only on events but on your underlying emotions. Think of it as the story of you and food. You can record your thoughts and feelings in your "Think Thin, Be Thin" notebook or computer file, or you can keep a separate journal. If you prefer, you can talk into a tape recorder, although seeing words in print has a more powerful subconscious impact.

Set aside a time and place to write. Many people prefer the end of the workday or before going to bed. You don't have to write every day, although we suggest three or four days a week. Try to write continuously for at least fifteen minutes. Don't worry about spelling or grammar or how much or how little you write. Remember that your words are for your eyes only. Don't censor yourself.

Stream-of-consciousness journaling

You might begin with stream-of-consciousness journaling and simply record whatever thoughts come into your mind. Sit quietly and breathe deeply. Once relaxed and settled, begin to write. Don't be surprised at the number and intensity of thoughts and feelings that emerge. As they become part of your awareness, they may lead to insights that have eluded you in the past. Psychologists believe that this happens because you are taking the time to hear what you are thinking.

If you run into writer's block, complete one of the following sentences:

When I think about my weight, I wish I had _____.

When I reflect on my eating habits, it seems _____.

Thinking about the way I treat my body, I feel _____.

Journaling for specific solutions

You also can use your journal to tackle specific issues and challenges.

- Write when you need to sort out complicated feelings about your weight or body image.

- Write when you're struggling to stay on your diet or when you stop working out.
- Write before going to dinner with friends to get ideas on how to manage the evening.
- Write afterward or the next day to chronicle the good choices you made or to note what you'll do differently the next time.

Reflective journaling

Try reflective journaling and write about yourself and your life in the third person. For example, you might write, "This morning as she lay in bed, she knew that she couldn't stand to live another day in her overweight body. She decided at that very moment to telephone her sister and ask . . ."

Dialogue journaling

You might experiment with dialogue journaling, in which you split yourself in two. In essence, you compose a script with two characters. One character might talk only of the benefits of losing weight. The other might complain about the drawbacks and difficulties. Write a back-and-forth conversation giving each character equal opportunity to make points and counterpoints.

There probably are at least 101 other ways of writing that may help you lose weight. We list several books on journaling in the recommended reading list in the Appendix. Experiment as much as you'd like and see what works best for you.

20

Reach Out for Support

Behind most successful dieters is a friend, spouse, buddy, coach, mentor, colleague, support group, or online community. According to a report from Purdue University, dieting women who teamed up with supportive partners lost as much as 30 percent more weight during a fifteen-month period than those who tried to do it alone.

Social support can take many forms but always involves having someone you can turn to and trust. Sometimes you can find all the support you need under your own roof: a parent, a sibling, a grown child, a spouse, or a combination. Ask directly for help, and feel free to make specific requests. Is your husband willing to watch the baby when you head for the gym? Would Mom not bake her all-too-delicious lasagna every week? Would your kids clean up after dinner so you can stay out of the kitchen? Also request positive feedback about how hard you're working or how good you look. The more applause you get, the more likely you are to stay the course.

A friend, coworker, or neighbor who also wants to lose weight can make a great diet buddy. Decide on a plan. Some diet partners compete to see who can lose five pounds first. Others switch off preparing meals and low-calorie snacks. You might walk or work out together, or check in with each other every evening, when you're most prone to overeating. Become comrades in arms and cheer each other on as the pounds come off.

21

Stage Your Exercise Program

Remember the five stages of change and your particular stage of motivational readiness for change (see Tip 3)? Here is a guide to the strategies most likely to help you activate an exercise program at your particular stage.

Precontemplation (not active and not thinking about becoming active)

• Set a small, reasonable goal that does not involve working up a sweat, such as standing rather than sitting when blow-drying your hair or doing squats while brushing your teeth.

Contemplation (not active but thinking about becoming active)

• Think back to activities you found enjoyable in the past. Did you ever rollerblade? Ice skate? Play softball? Row? Ask friends and coworkers if they can put you in touch with others with the same interest.

• List what you see as the cons of physical activity. For example, do you fear it will take up too much time? Write down three activities you could do if you woke up half an hour earlier or cut fifteen minutes off your lunch break.

• Determine the types of activity you can realistically

fit into your daily schedule. You might find a gym with child care in the morning, or sign up for an evening body-sculpting class.

• Find an image of the slimmer body you'd like to have—from a magazine advertisement, for example—and post it where you can see it often.

Preparation (active but not at recommended levels)

• Identify specific barriers that limit your activity. If you like to swim but the community pool closes for the winter, check out other facilities, such as a local Y. If you have a bad back or knee problems, consult a physical therapist for advice on safe exercises and exercises that may strengthen and protect your back or knees.

• Set specific daily and weekly goals. Your daily goal might begin with ten or fifteen minutes of activity and increase by five minutes every week or two. Your weekly goal might be to try a new activity, such as spinning or a dance class.

• Document your progress. You could use a monthly calendar to keep track of the number of days you've exercised as well as the length of each workout. Or you can keep a more detailed record, noting the types of exercise you do every day, the intensity you work at, the duration of each workout, etc.

Action (active at recommended levels for less than six months)

• Avoid boredom. Think through ways to vary your exercise routine. Take different routes on your walks. Invite different friends to join you. At the gym, alternate working with free weights and using resistance machines.

• Develop new athletic and sports skills. Try snowshoeing, kayaking, rock climbing, cardio-kickboxing, hip-hop dancing. Don't expect instant expertise. It usually takes four to six weeks to feel competent and get in the swing of a new activity.

• Intensify your effort. Increase your time or elevation on the treadmill, or do one more set (a certain number of repetitions) with your weights. As social scientists have demonstrated, extra effort reinforces and boosts your odds of reaching your goal.

22
As the World Grows Round

For the first time in history, the number of people who are too heavy is close to equaling the number who are too hungry: 1.1 billion of each, according to the Worldwatch Institute. "Globesity," as pundits call it, is an epidemic without borders. Seven in ten of the Dutch and Spanish, two in three Canadians, and one in two Britons, Germans, and Italians are overweight or obese. Obesity rates have quadrupled in Japan and are soaring in Latin America, where one in three Brazilians and four in ten Colombians are overweight. More than 115 million people in developing countries suffer from obesity-related problems.

America is second to none as a land of the large. The number of extremely obese adults—those at least a hundred pounds overweight—has quadrupled in the last two decades, to about 4 million. That works out to about one in every fifty men and women. How did so many get so fat?

• **Fattening lifestyle.** Bombarded by nonstop commercials for taste treats, tempted by foods in every form to munch and crunch, Americans are eating more—some 200 to 400 calories more a day than they did several decades ago. At the same time, experts estimate that most adults daily expend 200 to 300 fewer calories than people did twenty-five years ago.

• **Super-sized servings.** As the chart below shows, the size of many popular restaurant and packaged foods has increased two to five times during the past twenty years. According to studies of appetite and satiety, people presented with larger portions eat up to 30 percent more than they otherwise would.

Serving Sizes and How They've Grown in the Last 20 Years

	Then	Now	Caloric Difference
French fries	3.1 oz	3.6 oz	+68
Hamburger	5.7 oz	7 oz	+97
Soft drink	13.1 oz	19.9 oz	+49
Salty snack portions (pretzels, nuts, snack mix)	1 oz	1.6 oz	+93
Mexican dishes (burritos, tacos, enchiladas)	6.3 oz	8 oz	+133

• **More calories.** In the last thirty years, according to the Centers for Disease Control and Prevention (CDC), women have increased their caloric intake by 22 percent to an average of 1,877—considerably more than the CDC's recommended 1,600 calories for most women.

How can you pull away from the fattening crowd? Eat

incrementally less, and do incrementally more. Whether you're just starting a diet or have been on one for months, the following small changes can make a world of difference:

Have half a bagel rather than the whole thing.

Take the stairs instead of the elevator or escalator.

Order an open-faced sandwich instead of the standard two-slice.

Choose a hamburger instead of a cheeseburger.

Drink bottled water instead of juice.

Switch from blue cheese dressing to vinaigrette on your salad.

Have one glass of wine instead of two with dinner.

Add an extra ten minutes of activity to your day.

Play tennis for another twenty minutes.

23

Know Your Weights

Do you ease onto your scale, hoping for a certain number to appear—maybe what you weighed at age eighteen or before you had your first baby? If so, you may be setting yourself up for disappointment. Rather than focus on just one number, consider other ways to think about weight.

Dream weight   A weight you would choose if you could weigh whatever you wanted.

Happy weight   This weight is not the one you'd choose as your ideal, but you'd be happy if you weighed only this much.

Acceptable weight   A weight that would not make you particularly happy, but that you could be satisfied with.

Disappointed weight   A weight that would not be acceptable in any way.

Never-again weight   The all-time high you never
                        want to hit again.

In your notebook, jot down your dream weight, happy weight, acceptable weight, disappointed weight, and never-again weight. Then write down your actual weight, as of today.

How many pounds is your real weight from your acceptable weight?

Assuming you can lose a pound a week, how many weeks would it take you to get to that weight?

How do you envision yourself feeling and behaving once you reach your acceptable weight? Do you have any plans once you reach your acceptable weight, such as buying clothes or taking a weekend trip to see your college roommate? How will your life be different?

24

Automatic Thoughts, Automatic Failures

Every day you engage in an internal dialogue with yourself. The automatic thoughts that make up this self-talk may be part of the reason you're struggling to stay on your diet or can't keep off the weight you've lost. Train yourself to listen carefully and watch out for distorted ways of thinking:

All-or-nothing (dichotomous) thinking: Are your thoughts black and white, without any shades of gray? If the scale inches up by a pound or two, are you devastated? If it goes down, do you jump for joy?

Rather than going to extremes, remind yourself that scales don't tell the whole picture. You may weigh more simply because you're retaining water, or less because you've been sick. Next week you may be half a pound more or two pounds less.

Emotional reasoning: You prefer to feel rather than think. You tell yourself, "I don't 'feel' like dieting," or "I'm not 'in the mood' to exercise."

In this situation it doesn't matter how you feel. Use your brain, and do it anyway.

Fortunetelling: You don't think you can or ever will lose weight, so you wonder what's the use of even trying.

Rather than such doomsday forecasting, collect articles about people who have lost weight and kept it off. Cut out before-and-after pictures of people who have lost big and tape them on your refrigerator. Tell yourself, "If they can do it, so can I."

Personalizing and blaming: If it's too cold and icy for a walk, you blame the weather for ruining your workout plan. If your mother rewarded you with an extra dessert when you finished your homework, you hold her responsible for your being overweight twenty years later.

Get over it. Sooner or later, you have to take responsibility for your weight and well-being.

Overgeneralizing: You finish a single apple-cinnamon muffin and conclude that you've blown your diet.

Rather than exaggerating what you've done, work on developing a sense of perspective. Is consuming an extra 250 calories one day going to keep you from attaining your weight-loss goal?

This week listen carefully to how you think and how you talk to yourself. If you hear any of these self-defeating thoughts, turn them around or turn them off. Take your mind off automatic pilot and challenge yourself to think more logically.

25

Woman to Woman

More than 60 percent of adult U.S. women are overweight, and more than one third are obese. If you're among them, your excess pounds are hazardous to your health. When your diet determination wavers, read through this list to remind yourself of what you have to lose—and gain.

• **Arthritis.** Obese women have almost four times the risk of osteoarthritis as those who weigh less.

• **Breast cancer.** Women who gain twenty pounds or more after age eighteen are twice as likely to develop breast cancer after menopause than women who keep their weight fairly stable. Regardless of age, being overweight increases a woman's risk of inflammatory breast cancer, the most lethal form. Overweight women who develop breast cancer before menopause may have a shorter life span than thinner women with the same diagnosis. Weight gain after menopause may also increases breast cancer risk.

• **Endometrial cancer (cancer of the uterine lining).** Obese women have three to four times the risk of this malignancy than normal-weight women.

• **Cardiovascular disease.** As women become heavier,

they develop more risk factors for heart disease, including high blood pressure and high cholesterol.

• **Gallbladder disease.** Obese women have at least twice the risk of gallstones as women of normal weight.

• **Obstetric and gynecological complications.** Excess body fat can lead to menstrual irregularities and infertility. Overweight women who become pregnant are more prone to miscarriage, urinary-tract infection, high blood pressure, gestational diabetes, and other complications. They also experience longer labors, more cesarean deliveries, and more complications, such as infection, after childbirth.

• **Urinary stress incontinence.** Obesity is a well-documented risk factor for the involuntary loss of urine, especially after childbirth.

26

Your Top Ten Lists

In your notebook, write down ten things that are painful about being overweight. For instance:

- Not looking good in family photos
- Feeling embarrassed when seeing old friends from thinner days
- Struggling to bend over to tie shoes
- Calling in sick because you can't fit into any of your clothes
- Seeing people press themselves against the wall to make room for you to pass in the hallways

Now write ten things you could or would do if you were several sizes smaller. For example:

- Go inline skating with friends
- Wear a sexy little black dress
- Get in and out of the car more easily
- Post a photo on an online dating service
- Feel comfortable in shorts and a tank top

Record your two top ten lists in your notebook. Review your lists before you raid the refrigerator for that last piece of lemon meringue pie. Better yet, post your lists on the refrigerator. Each time you open the door, reflect on the disadvantages of weighing too much and the advantages of weighing less.

27
Use E-Prime

D o you know the most frequently used verb in the English language?

"To be" and all its various forms: am, is, are, was, were, be, been, being, will be, would be, might be.

Alfred Korzybski, founder of general semantics—the set of rules we use to derive meaning from words and sentences—identified two specific difficulties with the verb "to be." Both could affect your weight-loss efforts:

• **The *is* of identity.** For instance, if you say, "I *am* overweight," or "I *am* fat," you discount everything else about yourself and reinforce an identity that you plan to change. If you say, "I am on a diet," you set up an either/or frame of reference. You're either dieting or not. A better alternative: "I eat carefully and watch my food intake."

• **The *is* of predication.** In this case, if you say, "Watching my weight is impossible," you set up a self-fulfilling prophecy. You also distort reality since anyone, including you, can watch your weight.

Linguist David Bourland, Jr., a student of Korzybski's, developed a subset of the English language called E-prime that does not include the verb "to be." This innovative form of expression not only reduces the passive voice and removes generalizations but also eliminates distorted and all-or-nothing, either/or thinking.

We recommend experimenting with E-prime in order to set the stage for reaching your goal of lasting weight loss. Start with a practice sentence. Instead of "I'm fat," you might say, "I see myself as fat." Using "see" as a verb allows you to view fat as one of your characteristics but not the defining one.

As another option, you might say, "I carry too much weight on my body." This change in structure immediately transforms weight from a fixed personal characteristic to an object (weight) that requires your attention. This phrasing also invites you to take responsibility for your weight.

Ready to stretch your thinking further? Try eliminating the "to be" verb in the following sentences.

• My eating is out of control.
• I've always been overweight.
• Exercise isn't my thing.
• I'm a carb junkie.

Except for the examples, we wrote this entire entry in E-prime. Do the same the next few times you write in your notebook. This novel language may change more than your writing. By changing the way you think, define, and describe yourself, you can expect added resolve in your commitment to reaching your weight-loss goals.

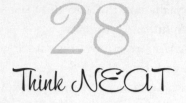

Think NEAT

D oes the carpet need vacuuming? Could a wood floor use some polishing? Is it time to weed the garden or rake the lawn?

These everyday chores carry an extra payoff: They burn calories through what scientists refer to as nonexercise activity thermogenesis, or NEAT. Even fidgeting can make a difference. In one experiment, volunteers of normal weight ate the same number of extra calories a day. Some gained weight. Others simply burned more calories, mostly by squirming, jiggling their feet as they sat, rolling their shoulders, and other minor movements. Fidgeting, researchers concluded, may be one of the ways the body naturally resists excess pounds.

NEAT is not an alternative to planned, purposeful exercise, but a convenient way to burn up even more calories so you push past a weight plateau and keep off the pounds you lose. Best of all, there are dozens of ways to become a NEAT-nik. Here are some ideas:

• Don't lie down when you can sit; don't sit when you can stand; don't stand when you can walk; don't walk when you can run.

• If you normally take the elevator to your office, walk the first five flights and then take the elevator. Coming down, walk the last ten flights.

• Play catch with your kids.

• If you have to wait for a delayed appointment, take a quick walk down the hall, around the building, or up a flight of stairs.

• Put extra oomph into your chores. Use wide, sweeping motions when you mop the floor. When unloading groceries, carry them into the house one bag at a time.

Boogie Calories Away

Activity	Calories per minute if you weigh			
	120 lb	140 lb	160 lb	180 lb
Bowling	1.2	1.4	1.6	1.9
Dancing	2.9	3.3	3.7	4.2
Gardening	5.0	5.9	6.7	7.5
Golf (with a cart)	2.1	2.5	2.8	3.2
Golf (pulling or carrying clubs)	4.6	5.4	6.2	7.0
Tennis	6.0	6.9	7.9	8.9

29

Get a Grip on Emotional Eating

O ccasionally all of us seek comfort at the tip of a spoon. However, many people use food as a way of coping with anger, frustration, stress, boredom, or fatigue. Whatever its motivation, emotional eating always involves eating for reasons other than physiological hunger. If you're not sure whether you do this, ask yourself the following questions:

- Do you eat when you're not hungry?
- Do you eat or continue eating even if the food doesn't taste good?
- Do you eat when you can't think of anything else to do?
- Do you eat when you're emotionally vulnerable—tired, frustrated, or worried?
- Do you eat after an argument or stressful situation to calm down?
- Do you eat as one of your favorite ways of enjoying yourself?
- Do you eat to reward yourself?
- Do you keep eating even after you're full?

Each "yes" answer indicates that you're eating in response to what you feel, not what you need. Diets may work for you, but the extra weight will inevitably creep back unless you confront your hidden motives for overeating. Since neither emotions nor food ever go away, you have to learn to deal with both for as long as you live.

To get a grip on your emotional eating, try our three-step plan:

Step 1: Know your triggers.

Whatever its specific motivation, emotional eating always involves eating for reasons other than physiological hunger. The key to getting it under control is awareness.

What are the feelings that set off an eating binge?

• Anger? Many women swallow their anger by eating because they're afraid of what might happen if they express it.

• Guilt? Some women eat because they feel they're always falling short as daughters, sisters, wives, or mothers.

• Rebellion? Eating may be the only way some women give themselves permission to take a break from being dutiful caregivers for others.

• Deprivation? At the end of a long day, a woman may justify turning to food as a well-deserved reward, maybe the first nice thing she's done for herself all day.

Did any of these possibilities hit home? If so, train yourself to take a step back and ask yourself a series of questions before you take a bite: Are you hungry? If not, what are you feeling? Stressed, tired, bored, anxious, sad, happy? Once you identify your true feelings, push deeper and ask why you feel this way. Try writing down your answers in your notebook. This is an even more effective way to help make sure that every bite you take is a conscious one.

Step 2: Put your body, not your emotions, in charge of what you eat.

To keep mind and body on an even keel, avoid getting so hungry and feeling so deprived that you become desperate and panicky. If you're facing an emotionally intense period—a corporate reorganization or a visit from an ornery relative—plan your meals and snacks in advance and try, as much as you can, to stick with your program. Rather than swearing off sweets forever, work indulgences into your weekly routine. If you plan to have a brownie for dessert on Friday night, you can look forward to it all week and not waste calories on a candy bar that won't taste as good.

Step 3: Focus on your feelings.

Let yourself feel how you're feeling without eating. Breathe deeply for a minute or two. Focus on the places in your body that feel tense. Rate the intensity of the emotion on a scale from ten (life or death) to one (truly trivial). Ask yourself: What's the worst-case scenario of feeling this way? Is food going to make it better in any way? Will it make it worse?

When you're tempted to eat but aren't hungry, write down the circumstances and try to discern the underlying reasons. If you eat ice cream at night, ask, "What does it get me?" The answer might be that it relaxes you. Once you realize that the ice cream is a means to an end, you can figure out something else you can do to get the same emotional benefits. If you're chronically frazzled, for instance, cut back on time demands. If you're lonely, sign up for a book club or evening class. If you're frustrated with your job, explore different career options.

What Are You Really Hungry For?

Is it a Hershey bar? Or a hug? Here's how to tell the difference between physical and emotional hunger:

Physical Hunger	Emotional Hunger
Builds gradually	Develops suddenly
Strikes below the neck (e.g., growling stomach)	Above the neck (e.g., a "taste" for ice cream)
Occurs several hours after a meal	Unrelated to time
Goes away when full	Persists despite fullness
Eating leads to feeling of satisfaction	Eating leads to guilt and shame

If you often eat to quell emotions, decide how you might tackle those feelings in a healthier way.

30
Become Mindful

Mindfulness is a modern form of an ancient Asian technique that involves maintaining awareness in the present moment. Mindfulness keeps you in the here-and-now, thinking about what *is* rather than *what if* or *if only.* You tune in to each part of your body, scanning from head to toe, noting the slightest sensation, and allowing whatever you experience—an itch, an ache, a feeling of warmth—to enter your awareness. Then you open yourself to focus on all the thoughts, sensations, sounds, and feelings that enter your awareness.

Medical researchers are experimenting with this approach to relieve stress, pain, and chronic health problems, such as migraines. Mindfulness can be particularly helpful in weight loss. When researchers compared obese women who practiced mindfulness with those in a control group, the mindful volunteers reported greater control of their eating and fewer binge-eating episodes. Here are some variations:

Controlled breathing
- Sit quietly in a room and focus on your breathing.
- Take five slow, deep breaths, pulling air down into

your lower abdomen. Concentrate on your breathing. If thoughts come into your mind, such as "I better check my messages," brush them aside and refocus on the rhythm of your breathing.

• As you breathe in, let your belly rise, and picture yourself inhaling warm, soothing air.

• As you breathe out, let your belly fall, and visualize yourself exhaling.

Gatha

Another variation is to use a gatha (a short poem, holy song, or psalm that keeps you focused on your life's meaning) along with mindful breathing. As you say the first line, breathe in. As you say the second line, breathe out. One of our favorite poems is:

> *Breathing in, I am calm and careful of what I eat,*
> *Breathing out, I feel in control of my eating.*

Feel free to change the words in any way you wish.

Walking meditation

This approach uses the rhythm of walking and breathing to stay in the present moment. As you walk, focus on your body. Be aware of your posture. Feel your feet hit the pavement or the treadmill. Feel your arms swing. Note your breathing. Keep your mind focused on the present. Don't allow yourself to get distracted by thoughts or sounds. Don't rehash conversations of the past or plan for the future. Walking meditation keeps you mindfully aware of your body. As your awareness grows, you'll feel more connected with your body, and you'll be less likely to abuse it with unhealthy eating.

Counting-breaths meditation

Focus on breathing and counting your breaths. If you have a few moments, try it now. Breathe smoothly in and out. Feel your diaphragm lift and fall as you count up to thirty. Whenever stress builds or the urge to overeat strikes, this technique can serve as a quick intervention.

31

United We Lose (Weight)

Do you know the most widely used form of psychotherapy today? Group therapy.

Rigorous studies have shown that groups are especially effective because they provide a safe and supportive environment where the members can share and discuss their problems, hear alternative ways to solve them, learn from the experiences of others, and discover new ways of interacting.

If you'd like to gain these benefits, start your own "Think Thin, Be Thin" weight-loss group. You don't need a professional to lead it. Tell your friends, neighbors, members of your community center, health club, church, book or investment club, and colleagues at work that you are looking for like-minded people to create a support group. Once others sign on (six to ten is ideal), decide where you'll meet and how often. Have a different person organize every meeting and set the agenda, make sure the group starts and stops on time, and keep the conversation on track. (Rotating this position builds group commitment and solidarity.)

Use the entries and exercises in *Think Thin, Be Thin* as topics of discussion. Make a pact to use several suggestions, and report your experiences at the next meeting. Try some exercises together, such as Tease Your Mind (see Tip 73) and I've Got a Secret (see Tip 96). If you already belong to Weight Watchers or another weight-loss group, introduce *Think Thin, Be Thin* to the members as an additional personal tool and group motivator.

Even if you don't consider yourself a joiner, you may discover unexpected advantages in banding together to take off pounds, including:

- empathy, support, and encouragement from individuals who truly understand what it's like to shop for a party dress with a slimmer friend or to hear a teenage daughter make an insensitive comment about her mother's weight
- greater awareness of your own distorted thinking and self-sabotaging comments
- collective problem solving
- accountability to both yourself and others
- laughter, intimacy, and friendship

32

Left Brain, Right Brain

What's your neurological style? Left brain or right brain? Although you routinely engage both sides of your brain, neuroscientists have found differences in the way certain tasks activate your left and right brain.

The left hemisphere is slightly more involved in logical, sequential, and analytical thinking. The right hemisphere tends to be more subjective, intuitive, and creative. When you're dieting, make the most of both: Feed your brain plenty of facts, but also involve your creativity and imagination.

Start with a job for your analytical side. In your "Think Thin, Be Thin" notebook or file, record the thirty foods you eat most often. Start with your favorite breakfast picks and work your way through the day. Beside each entry note the calories, protein, carbohydrates, and fat grams. You'll have them memorized within a week—and you'll be able to use the information the rest of your life.

Before you start cooking or go out for lunch, check your guide and calculate exactly what you'll be consuming. Then give the more imaginative part of your brain the job of conjuring up a picture of you in a tight-fitting pair of jeans. Visualize yourself struggling to get them up and over your thighs and hips. Then visualize yourself pulling them on with ease.

By using both sides of your brain, you'll find yourself making better food decisions.

33

Why You Sweat It

Starting an exercise program is the first step, but sticking with the routine can be just as challenging. According to studies of "exercise adherence," half of those who start working out drop out within six months.

To keep your muscles moving, engage your brain. According to research, the people most likely to continue an exercise program are those who keep the benefits in mind. In your first six months of working out, read the following list periodically to remind yourself of all you have to gain from thirty to sixty minutes of exercise most days of the week.

• **More life in your years—and more years in your life.** Physical activity slows the aging process, so you remain healthier and more active for a longer time. If you work out often and vigorously enough (a minimum of thirty minutes a day, six days a week), you can actually extend your life span.

• **Healthier heart.** Exercise increases the supply of oxygen to the heart, improves blood flow and cholesterol levels, and prevents blood clots. If your blood pressure isn't high, exercise will keep it under control. If it is elevated, regular exercise can bring it down to healthier levels.

• **Protection against cancer.** According to recent research moderate exercise, such as walking for half an hour most days, significantly reduces the risk of breast cancer—one of the few steps a woman can take to avoid this dreaded disease. Active people also have lower rates of colon and rectal cancer, possibly because exercise increases the rate at which waste moves through the digestive system.

• **Stronger bones.** Exercise, particularly strength training two or three times a week, increases bone density and lowers vulnerability to bone injury and weakness.

• **Better sleep.** Physical activity reduces stress chemicals and tension levels so you fall asleep faster, sleep longer, and wake up feeling more refreshed.

• **Brighter mood.** Exercise, which has proven as effective as medication in treating mild to moderate depression in numerous controlled studies (possibly because of its effects on brain chemistry), also increases energy, reduces anxiety, and boosts positive feelings. Regular exercise improves concentration and alertness at any age and significantly boosts cognitive functioning in older individuals.

• **Greater stamina.** As muscles become stronger, they function more smoothly so they can work longer and withstand more strain.

A bonus benefit: When you exercise regularly, you take control over one aspect of your life, which boosts your confidence in what else you can do, including lose weight.

34

How Rebellious Are You?

According to transactional analysis, conversations continually take place between three different aspects of your psyche: your Parent ego state, your Adult ego state, and your Child ego state.

The Parent ego state incorporates the thoughts, feelings, and actions that you observed in your parents or primary caretakers when growing up. When you are being judgmental, you are in your critical parent mode. When you are giving comfort and love, you are in your nurturing parent mode.

The Adult ego state gathers facts and information. It computes dispassionately, organizes information, and estimates outcomes much like a statistician would.

The Child ego state contains all the feelings and impulses that come with infancy and childhood. The Child is spontaneous, fun-loving, curious, creative, playful, and adaptive, as well as obstinate, rebellious, and hostile.

Each of these ego states affects the way you think, feel, and behave in many ways, including eating. For instance, when ordering lunch, you can "hear" the Parent, Adult, and Child in conversation.

Child: I think I'll order a double cheeseburger.

Adult: A double cheeseburger has 640 calories and 39 fat grams. A plain burger has 330 calories and 15 fat grams.

Rebellious Child: Who cares! I want to enjoy lunch and not think about dieting.

Nurturing Parent: Maybe a plain burger would be better and you'd save yourself a lot of calories.

Adaptive Child: Okay, I guess I'll have a plain burger.

Nurturing Parent: Good decision.

That may end the discussion, or your Rebellious Child may declare, "Oh, who cares. I'm ordering a double cheeseburger, fries, and a shake. I deserve it."

Here's another example.

Parent: This would be a great day to take a walk and get some exercise.

Adult: You've been sitting at the computer all day and haven't done anything physical.

Rebellious Child: Walking is boring. And I hate exercise.

Nurturing Parent: It's a beautiful day and you'll feel good once you get out in the fresh air.

Adaptive, Creative Child: Yeah, okay. I'll call Lisa and see if she can walk with me. Then we can run to the mall and I can get that new lipstick I saw advertised.

Recognizing the interactions between your Parent, Adult, and Child can help you understand how you can be conscientious about your diet and determined to exercise one minute, then blow your diet and skip exercise the next.

The following exercise uses transactional analysis to provide insight into your weight-loss struggles.

Your book club is having a dessert extravaganza to celebrate the holidays, and each member is bringing a dessert from countries in the books you've read. After ten months of dieting, you've lost thirty-two pounds and are determined to reach your weight-loss goal. As you are driving to your book club meeting, what would you hear from:

- Your Parent, being nurturing and being critical?
- Your Adult?
- Your Child, being rebellious, being adaptive?

If you find your Rebellious Child exerting too much power, try to reinforce your Nurturing Parent and keep telling yourself, "You can do what you set your mind to do. You have great strength. Staying on your diet and working out are two of the best choices you can make."

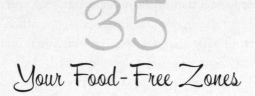

35
Your Food-Free Zones

If you want help in controlling how much you eat, enforce some environmental controls on where you eat. Start by looking over the list, deciding where you are most likely to eat.

_____ at the kitchen table
_____ at the dining room table
_____ at the kitchen counter
_____ standing in front of the refrigerator
_____ in a fast-food restaurant
_____ in a cafeteria or lunchroom
_____ in a car, train, or bus
_____ at your desk
_____ in front of the television
_____ in bed
_____ at a restaurant
_____ at friends' homes
_____ at sporting or social events
_____ other places, such as _____

Of the places you found you are most likely to eat, which might become no-eating zones?

We suggest a ban on food any place that you sleep or work. This eliminates the bedroom and office. Several weeks from now, expand your no-food territory to the places you read, watch television, or talk on the phone. Declare your car (or at least the driver's seat) a no-food zone. Make your designated dining areas as small as possible—not the entire kitchen, but the kitchen table, for instance. Anytime you want to eat at home, head for your designated dining destination, even if it's only to munch some chips or a bunch of grapes. This makes you more aware of everything you're putting in your mouth—and gives you time to think and reconsider if you really want a snack.

36
Five Key Questions

Often a therapist asks carefully crafted questions in order to bring forth or access information from the unconscious—the thoughts and feelings that are not part of your conscious awareness. The following five questions, examples of this approach, are not casual inquiries, but keys to understanding the roots of your weight problem. Although these questions may seem simple at first glance, give yourself time to answer them fully. Be as introspective as possible. We suggest recording your answers in your "Think Thin, Be Thin" notebook or file because seeing your thoughts leads to deeper reflection and insight.

1. What are the advantages of being overweight?

At first, you may wonder what possible advantage could come from being overweight. Therapists, however, believe that all behavior serves a purpose. Even destructive behaviors such as overeating, gaining fifty pounds, or not working out have a hidden benefit. You may not understand why you've allowed yourself to overeat and gain weight. But on an unconscious level, these behaviors provide some advantages.

By answering this first question, you may find that you use your weight to justify why you don't have a boyfriend or you didn't get the promotion you expected. Maybe being overweight allows you to put off certain goals, such as changing jobs, taking a dance class with your friends, or traveling abroad. Or it might simply provide the excuse you need to stay home and read, rather than go to events where you feel self-conscious.

2. *How did you acquire your current shape?*

This question may make you realize that you started putting on pounds in college or after your last pregnancy. Maybe you gained weight after a bad breakup or a divorce. Or maybe years of poor eating habits, such as fast-food lunches or late-night snacks, finally caught up with you.

Figuring out when and how you put on weight helps in two ways. You become more forgiving of your current weight because you understand its origins. You also distance yourself from your weight, which allows you to see it as just another challenge in life.

3. *What are the negative consequences of not changing your weight?*

Will you continue to feel unattractive or suffer from low self-esteem? Will you worry about never getting married or having a baby? Will you feel uncomfortable making love? This question helps you explore something you may avoid: the disadvantages of continuing to be overweight. Realizing where you're headed can provide greater incentive for changing direction.

4. What are you doing about your weight?

Even though you want to lose weight, you may not be doing much except thinking about it. Or you may have answered that you are using an affirmation, keeping a food diary, and cutting down on sweets. Answering this question comprehensively can move you from the contemplation to the action stage of change. If you're already working on your weight, the answer can boost your motivation to stay the course.

5. What rewards will you gain if you change?

Becoming fit and healthy may be its own reward, but you probably envision more returns on the time and energy you invest in weight loss. These might include feeling sexier, buying new clothes, switching careers, lowering your risk of health problems, or simply liking yourself again. As you think about all that you can gain, you will be more motivated to lose.

This exercise in introspection can help at any stage of a weight-loss program. Your answers and perspective will shift as you make progress toward your goals. If you get stuck or discouraged along the way, these questions can put you in touch with your unconscious wishes and worries.

37

A Night at the Movies

C an watching a movie help you lose weight?
Yes, if you choose the right film—and skip the popcorn.

Therapists often recommend movies as an "adjunctive" or supplemental approach that can help individuals solve their problems and reach their goals. Although books can provide information on why you should change, movies, which often elicit more powerful feelings, can motivate you to follow through.

The following movies provide not only a good deal of laughter but inspiration and encouragement as well.

• *As Good as It Gets* (1997) PG-13. Melvin Udall, played by actor Jack Nicholson, suffers from obsessive-compulsive disorder. Refusing to let anyone serve him at the local neighborhood restaurant except waitress Carol Connelly (Helen Hunt), he reluctantly falls in love with her. Little by little, he makes adjustments in his daily behaviors. He learns to look beyond himself and see that others need nurturing, love, and emotional support.

• *Groundhog Day* (1993) PG. A television weatherman (Bill Murray) sent to cover the annual Groundhog Day ceremony in Punxsutawney, Pennsylvania, gets caught in a time warp and must repeat the day over and over until he gets the day "right" and becomes less selfish and self-absorbed. With each replay of February 2, Murray transforms himself into a more thoughtful, generous, seize-the-day type of guy.

• *The Full Monty* (1997), R. In order to make money, a group of unemployed steelworkers in Sheffield, England, decide to become male strippers. As the story unfolds, each character sets his priorities and resolves to make more of life. This movie also underscores the idea that most problems are solvable if you don't give up.

• *What About Bob?* (1991), PG. Bob (Bill Murray) attaches himself to his psychiatrist (Richard Dreyfuss), who urges him to take "baby steps" to overcome his emotional disabilities. The outrageous and outrageously funny story line reminds us that life is filled with twists and turns, struggles and triumphs. The best course of action, despite all odds, is to keep moving forward in a positive direction.

38

Rx: Relax

Rather than reaching for food to soothe yourself, master a relaxation technique. One of the most effective is progressive relaxation, which involves intentionally increasing and then decreasing tension in the muscles. Relaxing your muscles can quiet the mind, restore internal balance, and lower stress, which can prevent emotional eating.

Here are some basic guidelines:

• Sit quietly in a comfortable position.

• Close your eyes.

• Breathe through your nose. Focus on your breaths. At the end of each exhalation, say the word "one" silently to yourself, establishing the following pattern: Breathe in . . . out, "one"; in . . . out, "one." Breathe easily and naturally.

• Deeply clench and then relax various muscles, beginning with the hands and proceeding to the arms, shoulders, neck, face, chest, stomach, and down each leg to the toes.

• Do not worry about achieving a deep level of relaxation in your first tries. Permit relaxation to occur at its own pace. When distracting thoughts flit into your mind, dismiss them and return to repeating the word "one."

With practice, you will be able to reach a state of relaxation with little effort.

• Continue this exercise for ten to twenty minutes. You may open your eyes to check the time, but do not use an alarm clock, which may startle you by its ring. When you finish, sit quietly for several minutes, at first with your eyes closed and then with them open. Wait a few minutes before standing up.

Try to give yourself the pleasure of progressive relaxation each day and you'll find food simply won't take on more emotional importance than it deserves.

39

Are You Too Defensive?

When feeling anxious, we all rely on defense mechanisms, which are unconscious ways of suppressing unpleasant thoughts and impulses. Because weight issues generate so much anxiety, you may be using your defense mechanisms in ways that sabotage your goals. Here are some examples:

• **Repression:** Forgetting or ejecting ideas or information from conscious awareness. For instance, you might read an article that obese women are more likely to get breast cancer and not remember any of the information several minutes later.

• **Rationalization:** Substituting "good," acceptable reasons for the real motivations for your behavior. For example, you take an extra large slice of homemade pie and tell yourself you're showing your hostess how much you appreciate her baking.

• **Displacement:** Redirecting or transferring thoughts and behavior from one object or person to another. While you may be upset at your mother for commenting about your weight, you snap at your husband rather than discussing it with her.

• **Projection:** Attributing your own undesirable characteristics to others. "Everyone eats too much at buffets,"
you might say, as you load your plate for the third time.

• **Denial:** Refusal to believe information or the true nature of a threat. Even if your doctor cautions you about
your weight and high cholesterol, you might say to yourself, "I'm only thirty-three. I'm too young to worry about
a heart attack."

Read through the list of defense mechanisms again,
and jot down in your journal examples of how you may
be using them to avoid dealing with your weight. Becoming consciously aware of how you "defend" your weight
moves you closer to losing extra pounds.

40

Count the Ways

Take an inventory of a hundred things you like about yourself, and list them in your "Think Thin, Be Thin" notebook or computer file. Don't hesitate to blow your own horn as you remind yourself of the qualities that make you unique and valuable.

Here are some ideas to get you going:

- I am a loyal friend.
- I have a great sense of humor.
- I roll with the punches.
- I try to do my best at everything I undertake.
- I tell terrific ghost stories.
- I have a knack for putting people at ease.

Add to your list over several days or weeks. Once you complete it, keep a copy on your nightstand, on your kitchen counter, or post it on the refrigerator. Glance at it often. When you're feeling down or unappreciated, don't seek solace from a chocolate bar. Read your list instead. Seeing your good qualities in print is amazingly uplifting. As studies confirm, the better you feel about yourself, the less likely you are to turn to food for comfort.

41

Tap, Tap, Tap Your Appetite Away

Are you about to head for the fridge or vending machine because you feel anxious and think a snack would make you feel better? Instead try tapping on some of your body's acupuncture meridians. This exercise, modified from an unorthodox approach called Thought Field Therapy draws on ancient Chinese theories of energy flow. Tapping on specific sites on your body, and using a specific sequence, allows you to unblock and realign the flow of energy. Here's how to give it a try:

1. Take your right or left hand and put two or three fingers on the bony ridge at the far corner of one of your eyes, and tap gently ten times on the spot.
2. Put your fingers under one of your armpits. Slide them down about three or four inches until you feel a slight indentation. Tap gently ten times where you feel the indentation.
3. Take your fingers and place them on the indentation between your collarbones, right where a bow tie would sit. Now move your fingers about four inches down and then to the left about four inches, a little

above your heart. Again, you should feel a slight indentation. Tap gently ten times.

4. Stretch out the fingers of one of your hands, and between your baby finger and your ring finger, start tapping. As you're tapping, do the following:

> *Close your eyes.*
> *Open your eyes wide.*
> *Look down to the right without moving your head.*
> *Look down to the left without moving your head.*
> *Roll your eyes in a circle to the right.*
> *Roll your eyes in a circle to the left.*
> *Hum a short tune out loud, about five or six notes. (Re-*
> *member to keep tapping.)*
> *Count to five out loud.*
> *Again, hum five or six notes of a short tune.*

After following the directions a half-dozen times,
you'll have them memorized. You can do this tapping sequence almost anywhere. Although this exercise may seem
bizarre and remains largely untested, many therapists report that it helps clients reduce tension and the desire
to eat.

42

"Chunking"

Who wants to chunk up?
Before you answer, let us explain that we are not talking about being thickly set, but about the way you think, process thoughts, and communicate.

Chunking is a term from the psychological approach called neurolinguistic programming (NLP). "Neuro" refers to the brain and the neural networks that feed it information. "Linguistic" refers to the verbal and nonverbal messages that flow through the neural pathways. Programming converts these messages into thoughts and behaviors. By using NLP, you can learn to create and manipulate thoughts, visualize a desired outcome, and move closer to your weight-loss goal. Along the way you will literally change your brain.

"Chunking up" means moving from the specific to the general in order to communicate on a more abstract level. This allows you to see the bigger picture. "Chunking down" means moving from the general to the specific so you communicate in more detail. Both ways of communicating can set the stage for change—chunking up, by giving you a broader perspective on the problem; chunking down, by allowing you to look more closely.

Chunking Up

"What purpose does that have?"

This is the key question in chunking up. Although it may sound stilted, it forces your brain to step up and provide more and more information. The following example illustrates how this works in psychotherapy:

Molly, who is struggling to lose weight, can see only the negative aspects of being overweight. She starts the conversation by saying, "I can't get into any of my clothes."

The therapist asks, "What purpose does that have?"

Molly responds, "I don't have anything to wear when it's time to go out."

The therapist asks, "What purpose does that have?"

Molly says, "It allows me to stay home."

The therapist asks, "What purpose does that have?"

Molly says, "I don't like being in social situations. Deep down I'm afraid of what people think."

The therapist asks, "What purpose does that have?"

Molly says, "It gives me a reason to feel sorry for myself."

As the therapist repeats the question, Molly realizes that her excess weight, although upsetting on a conscious level, provides some secondary rewards, such as an excuse to avoid uncomfortable social situations and a reason to feel sorry for herself.

By continuing to use the question, "What purpose does that have?" Molly and her therapist can uncover other reasons she unconsciously might be holding on to her weight. Once Molly becomes aware of them, she will be better able to become and stay slim.

Chunking Down

In going from the general to the specific, the key NLP question is, "What provides an example of that?"

This time Molly says, "I really need to lose weight."

The therapist asks, "What provides an example of that?"

Molly says, "I can't get into any of my clothes."

The therapist asks, "What provides an example of that?"

Molly responds, "I can't zip my pants or button my blouses."

By focusing on details, Molly becomes aware of how much weight she has put on and sees her weight problem more clearly and vividly.

Whether you chunk up or down, seeing things from a different perspective and becoming aware of information that may have eluded you can set the wheels of change in motion.

Copy the following comments in your "Think Thin, Be Thin" notebook or file. Then try chunking up and down with each comment:

"No matter how hard I try I can't seem to stay on my diet."

"I don't have the time to exercise."

"I can't stand all the weight I've gained."

Change Your Body Language

Although words are mighty, more than 90 percent of communication is nonverbal. While we speak with our vocal cords, we express ourselves with our facial expressions, tone of voice, gestures, and posture. We may raise our voices when angry, fold our arms in front of our chests defensively, or let our shoulders sag when sad or weary.

Read the messages your body is sending right now:

- How are you standing or sitting?
- Are you slumping, with your shoulders forward and your chin down? Or are your shoulders back and chin up?
- How about your stomach? Is it pouching out, or are you pulling it in?

Slumping shoulders, a dropped chin, and a sagging belly suggest weariness and defeatism. Standing straight, pulling your shoulders back, lifting your chin, and sucking in your stomach show that you're in control and ready for action.

As an experiment, try both these postures now. First slouch, then sit or stand tall. Which posture makes you feel you can shape up and tackle your weight? The answer is obvious. Walk around all day with your stomach in and your shoulders back. Let your body language remind you to take charge of the way you look and feel.

44

Mind Over Platter

Behavioral psychologists have found that manipulating various environmental cues—sounds, sights, sensations, settings—can affect how test subjects, be they animal or human, respond to food. By changing your eating environmental cues, you can change your eating patterns.

• **Plate theory.** Even if you're having only a few crackers or carrots, feed yourself the way you'd serve a guest—with real dishes and silverware. This transforms every eating episode into a dining experience that engages mind as well as mouth. Trade in the typical 10½-inch dinner plate for an 8¼-inch plate. At a buffet, use only a smaller salad or dessert plate. According to obesity experts, switching to a smaller plate may reduce the amount of food you put on your plate by 20 percent because your eyes read the plate as full.

• **Dine by candlelight.** In various studies, volunteers ate less food when blindfolded, but they felt just as full as usual. Why? Scientists theorize that without vision, individuals had to rely on internal signals of hunger and satisfaction, messages usually overwhelmed by other sources of stimulation. Other experiments have shown that people eat more food when it is placed under bright light, such as at an eat-all-you-can buffet. If you can't dim the lights, close your eyes every now and then as you eat just to tune in to your body's internal messages.

• **Eat to the beat.** Turning on soothing music when you eat may help you chew slower and eat less. In a study at Johns Hopkins University, volunteers ate with various musical backgrounds for a month. In silence they averaged 3.9 bites per minute and finished eating in about 40 minutes; one third asked for seconds. With lively music, their mouths moved more quickly, up to 5.1 bites per minute; they finished eating in just 31 minutes, and about half asked for another helping. But with slow, restful tunes, volunteers took fewer and smaller bites, chewed longer and more slowly, and extended their eating time to almost sixty minutes. Most didn't even finish their first serving, yet they reported feeling fuller and more satisfied than after eating to a faster tune.

• **"The End."** When these words flash on the screen, you know the movie's over. Train your taste buds to recognize the end of a meal or snack. Brush your teeth right after dinner; bring mints with you if you go out to eat. Anything with a fresh taste, such as breath mints, gum, or toothpaste, will signal your brain that you're done eating. And since you eliminate the taste of your meal or snack, you won't want more of the food you were just eating.

45

Meditation

Imagine a therapy that relieves stress, lowers blood pressure, helps control pain, decreases anxiety, lifts depression, reduces hostility, elevates consciousness, and creates a sense of harmony and well-being.

There is such a treatment: meditation. It's been used in myriad forms for centuries, and more than five hundred scientific studies have confirmed its benefits. We also have new understanding of why meditation works. As neuro-imaging scans reveal, it activates the sections of the brain in charge of the autonomic nervous system, which governs bodily functions, such as digestion and blood pressure, that we cannot consciously control.

Maybe you're already among the estimated 10 million Americans who meditate regularly. If not, we suggest you start. Meditation can strengthen your self-awareness, which will help you think more positively about yourself, feel in greater control over the choices you make, and see the future in more optimistic terms—three essentials for successful weight loss and management.

The various forms of meditation have several common elements: sitting quietly for fifteen or twenty minutes once or twice a day, concentrating on a word or image, and breathing slowly and rhythmically.

In transcendental meditation, the meditator repeats a mantra or special phrase. One popular mantra is Om, which refers to the source of all light, love, and wisdom. Mahatma Gandhi's mantra was Rama, Rama, meaning "he who fills us with abiding joy." Because you're trying to lose weight, you might chose a relevant word from another language, such as *magro* or *magra*, the Italian adjective (masculine and feminine, respectively) for thin, or *embamba*, which means thin in Swahili. Or make up a word of your own.

Once you choose your mantra, stick with it. As you sit quietly and breathe, concentrate on your mantra, which you can repeat under your breath, silently in your head, or out loud. You also can use your mantra when you're not meditating. Repeat it as you walk or fold laundry. If you're tempted to eat something you know you shouldn't, call on your mantra. It will calm you and refocus your thoughts.

Another option is reflective meditation, which focuses your thoughts on how a problem first developed, and the additional difficulties it presents. As you sit, breathe in and out, relax, and reflect on your difficulties with your weight. When did it first become an issue? In early adolescence? After a cross-country move? When you had your second child? When you turned forty? Try to identify something in your life that your extra weight is helping you avoid, such as dating or applying for a transfer or promotion. Or perhaps it's your excuse to stay inactive or avoid going on a family cruise. Then turn your thoughts to some good that's come from being overweight, such as meeting a wonderful friend in a weight-loss group or developing a closer relationship with your daughter-in-law as the two of you exchange low-cal recipes. Continue your reflections over several weeks. As you thoughtfully reflect on your weight issue, expect to gain a greater understanding of how your weight plays a more significant role in your life than you may have imagined.

46

Stop Giving Yourself Orders

D o you have a voice inside that issues orders and barks criticisms like a drill sergeant? As we explained in Tip 15, negative thoughts can do more harm than good. The same is true with commands. Using "should" words creates stress, which can trigger further eating. For example, saying to yourself, "I should go on a diet," or "I ought to lose weight," invites you to feel more overwhelmed and anxious.

Should and ought words also set up an internal critical parent/rebellious child scenario similar to the one described in Tip 34. As the critical parent, you tell yourself what to do: for example, "You need to lose weight." As the rebellious child, you eat three desserts.

If shoulds and oughts fill your self-talk, write out a have-to list of things you tell yourself about your health, weight, and lifestyle. For example, "I have to stop eating jelly doughnuts every morning," or "I have to give up corn chips."

In your notebook write five items beginning with "I have to."

Next rewrite your list, but instead of using the words "I have to," use the words "I choose to."

Replacing the words "I have to" with "I choose to" moves you from helplessness to a position of power.

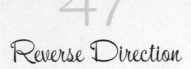

47

Reverse Direction

If you feel trapped in a diet rut, try turning some tactics around:

• **Track what you don't eat.** Rather than log every morsel that crosses your lips, record what didn't make its way into your mouth. We call this technique "food reversal." Focus on the half of the muffin you left behind at breakfast; the soft drink you decided not to order at lunch, the spice cookies you passed up at the office. Each day grow your list. Feel the gratification of adding to it instead of fretting over everything you might have recorded in a regular food diary.

• **Reverse your daily eating pattern.** If you, like many women, tend to skip breakfast, have a light lunch, and then graze all evening, shift your schedule so you consume the bulk of your calories before 4:00 p.m. In a classic experiment at the University of Minnesota, seven volunteers ate one 2,000-calorie meal a day for two weeks. During the first week, they ate at 7:00 a.m.; during the second, at 5:30 p.m. When breakfast was their only meal, they all lost weight: 1.25 pounds on average. When they ate only in the late afternoon, every person except one gained almost a pound.

48

Feed Your Soul

"If prayer were available in pill form, no pharmacy could stock enough of it," says internist Dale Matthews, M.D., author of *The Faith Factor*, who estimates that about 75 percent of studies of the impact of spiritual practices, such as regular prayer, have confirmed health benefits. Even when age, health, habits, socioeconomics, and other factors are considered, individuals who pray regularly and attend religious services stay healthier and live longer than those who rarely or never do.

One reason, suggests psychiatrist Harold Koenig, M.D., of Duke University Medical Center, is that people who engage in religious practices have a "perception of control" that strengthens their resolve, as opposed to a "perception of helplessness" that weakens it. Faith in a higher power promotes a positive outlook, optimism, healthy behavior, and a sense of self-efficacy—all essential for weight-loss success.

Although you can't simply pray pounds away, here are some suggestions that can feed your spirit—and keep you from overfeeding your body:

• If you are religious, deepen your spiritual commitment through prayer, more frequent church attendance, or joining a prayer group. Pray regularly with your family. Read Scriptures, chant in the Buddhist tradition, or say the rosary. As you nourish your spiritual side, you will feel greater serenity and control, including control of your eating.

• If you are not religious, meditate (see Tip 45) and read the writings of inspired people of deep faith, such as Rabbi Harold Kushner and the Rev. Martin Luther King, Jr.

• Perform acts of selfless service. Volunteer at a hospital or retirement home. Work in a literacy program. Become a platelet donor for the American Red Cross or a driver for Meals on Wheels. When people give to others, they develop a stronger sense of self-worth, which leads to positive lifestyle changes.

• Ask yourself, "What is my higher value?" Your higher value is your ultimate goal, what you most want to accomplish. When you're tempted to take a second helping, ask yourself, "What is my higher value?" Is it to lose weight, feel better, and eat healthier—or to give in to your immediate desire? When you're feeling too weary to swim laps, ask yourself, "What is my higher value?" Is it to crash on the sofa every evening or to keep your body healthy and fit?

49

Choose to Control Your Cravings

Eating is a necessity, but each bite you take is a choice. Even cravings that seem uncontrollable are within your power to choose. The secret: Engage your brain, and prepare a plan to thwart temptation.

• **Take a sip.** Many people misinterpret cravings for fluid as food cravings and eat to satisfy their thirst. To wash away such cravings, take frequent sips of small amounts of water (three to four ounces) rather than gulping a large glass straight down. (The activity itself distracts you from your craving.) If it's fluid your body really needs, you should soon forget you wanted to eat.

• **Take ten.** Rather than indulge yourself immediately, check the time and wait a full ten minutes before giving in to a craving. Put the ice cream back in the freezer or the candy bar back on the shelf. Walk away, and busy yourself with work or chores. More often than not, the craving will pass.

• **If you're a junk-food junkie.** If you eat fast food every day, switch to every other day, then every three days, then once a week. Order only one item, such as popcorn chicken, rather than a complete meal. Eat fruit half an hour before going to the drive-in window or restaurant. Drink water, coffee, or iced tea, rather than a milk shake.

• **Try the "bait and switch."** When you get a craving, go ahead and satisfy it, but with a slimmer substitute. Here are some examples:

When you want	Switch to
Chocolate ice cream: 8 ounces = 320 calories	Fat-free chocolate ice cream: 8 ounces = 90 calories
	Yogurt: 8 ounces = 100 calories
French fries: large = 535 calories	Baked potato = 250 calories
Fried chicken = 495 calories	Roasted chicken (without skin) = 250 calories
Bacon (3 slices) and two eggs = 400 calories	Deli-style ham (2 slices) and egg substitutes = 100 calories
Hot dog = 180 calories	Light hot dog (95% fat-free) = 55 calories, or turkey dog = 40 calories

• **The cold-turkey cure.** To overcome a craving that seems beyond control, such as a chocolate addiction, go without the food you adore for twelve weeks. Tell yourself that anyone can get through anything for twelve weeks. After that, the craving will ease. In time you'll be able to have one piece of chocolate, rather than the whole box.

50

From Fat to Fit

What is the first recommendation of the diet doctors who head weight-management programs at leading medical centers?

Become as fit as you can be at the weight you are.

Overweight people who exercise regularly are at less risk of serious health risks than both inactive heavy individuals and leaner sedentary folks. In a twenty-five-year study of more than 25,000 mainly middle-aged men, those who were fat but fit were nearly three times less likely to die at an early age than unfit obese men. Other research suggests that the same is true for women.

Going from fat to fit isn't a quick or easy process. But whatever your weight or fitness level, you can start where you are and move forward.

Although no exercise or fitness plan suits everybody at every age and stage of life, sports medicine specialists recommend the F.I.T.T. formula (for frequency, intensity, time, and type):

Frequency: How often do you exercise?

Face it: A Saturday-morning hike or an hour at the gym every week won't whip you into shape. You need to exercise more often to reap the benefit. Federal health officials, such as the Surgeon General's office, recommend a minimum of three to five days of aerobic or cardiovascular training and two days of resistance and flexibility training.

Intensity: How hard do you work out?

Whether you're doing an aerobic exercise or working on muscle strength, you need to meet a greater-than-normal challenge. If you're walking or running, move fast enough to speed up your heart rate. Start with a 15-minute walk or jog, and increase time and distance gradually as you go farther and faster. For strength training, you can increase the amount of weight you lift, the resistance you work against, or the number of repetitions.

Time: How long should you work out?

The answer depends on how hard you're working. If you're exercising at high intensity (such as biking uphill or jogging at a 10-minute-a-mile pace), you don't need to continue as long as when you're gliding down hills or walking at a slower pace. For strength and flexibility training, pay attention to the number of repetitions of doing chest presses or doing biceps curls rather than total time.

Type: What kind of exercise are you doing?

Ideally, your weekly workouts should include a mix of aerobic activities, strength training, and flexibility exercises. Consider all the options you have for becoming fitter and slimmer, and choose those you enjoy most. If you hate running, try cycling or spinning. If you feel uncomfortable at a gym or health club, buy a workout video or DVD and exercise at home, or ask a friend to start walking with you in the morning.

EXERCISE OPTIONS
Aerobic (cardiovascular):

Walking / hiking

Jogging / running

Swimming

Biking

Spinning

Kayaking / canoeing

Dance

Tennis

Handball

Cross-country skiing

Basketball

Soccer

Skipping rope

Step training or bench aerobics

Stair climbing

Cardio-kickboxing

Strength training

Free weights

Resistance machines

Body-sculpting classes

Rock or wall climbing

Circuit training

Weighted pulleys

Flexibility / Coordination

Stretching

Pilates

Yoga

Fitball classes (exercises with a large inflated ball)

Tai chi

51

Learn from Your Past

In your "Think Thin, Be Thin" notebook or file, list twelve of your achievements, from childhood to now. You might include everything from your first piano recital, to becoming a cheerleader in high school, to getting your real-estate license. Under each achievement, record three things that made it possible. For example:

Making the cheerleading squad in high school

- Six years of gymnastics
- Nightly practice with the squad for four months before making the team
- Weekend practices with friends at home

Getting your real-estate license

- Taking evening courses
- Doing grunt work, like posting Open House signs
- Studying every weekend for months to pass the licensing test

In both these examples, the prerequisites to success were practice and hard work. Look over your achievements, and identify the steps that led to each one.

How can you apply the same principles to your weight-loss goals so history can repeat itself? Jot some ideas in your notebook.

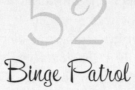

Binge Patrol

About 2 percent of Americans may be binge eaters. You're more likely to binge if you're young and female. Not all binge eaters are fat, but they get fat if they continue this unhealthy behavior.

Although everyone overeats on occasion, a binge is more extreme. You know you're on a binge if you experience at least three of the following:

- Eating much more rapidly than usual
- Eating until you feel uncomfortably full
- Eating large amounts of food when not feeling physically hungry
- Eating large amounts of food in a limited period of time
- Eating alone because you're embarrassed by what, how, and how much you eat

In the course of several hours, binge eaters may consume 2,000 or more calories—more than many people eat in a day. After binges, they usually do not induce vomiting, use laxatives, or rely on other means, such as fasting, to control weight. They simply get fatter. As their weight climbs, they become depressed, anxious, or troubled by more psychological symptoms than others of comparable weight.

If you occasionally go on eating binges, use the behavioral technique called "habit reversal," and replace your bingeing with a competing behavior. For example, every time you're tempted to binge, immediately do something else. Play the piano, give yourself a manicure, jump on the treadmill, or e-mail us or your diet buddy about your day. Do anything that keeps food out of your mouth.

If you binge twice a week or more for at least a six-month period, you may have binge-eating disorder, which may require professional help. Treatment usually consists of cognitive-behavioral therapy, either individually or in a group setting. As chronic binge eaters recognize their unhealthy behavior and confront the underlying issues, they usually are able to stop bingeing and resume normal eating patterns.

53

The Bowery El Effect

Years ago a noisy elevated train ran along Third Avenue in New York City. Soon after the line closed, people began reporting strange noises at about the times the train used to rumble through the neighborhood. The New Yorkers were "hearing" the familiar noise of the train. This phenomenon was later termed "the Bowery El effect."

We all carry a model of the world encoded in our brains. If the input you receive and your model of the world agrees, everything feels right. But when something changes, things don't feel the same, and you may unconsciously try to re-create the way things were.

As you continue to make changes in order to lose weight, you can expect to feel the Bowery El effect. If you always order a large soda, popcorn, and a box of Raisinettes when you go to a movie, the next time you go to the theater, things may not seem quite right without them. You may not even enjoy the movie as much.

Habit reversal, the behavioral technique described in the preceding tip, can ease the transition from old, familiar ways to new ones. Consciously adopt a new behavior to replace your previous habit. For example, bring bottled water and some grapes to the movie. If you used to watch television and snack all evening, sign up for a yoga or stretch class at the gym or a lecture series at a museum. Within a few weeks, your new behavior will become routine, and you'll no longer hear the echoes of the Bowery El.

54

Love the Body You're In

When women look in the mirror, they usually don't like what they see. Even those with a healthy body mass index (BMI) generally don't feel satisfied with their weight. Most want to drop to 90 percent of the "ideal" for their height.

This isn't surprising. We are surrounded by idealized images of female bodies that bear little resemblance to the way most women look. Over the past several decades, the media's notion of the ideal female form has shrunk. Women in *Playboy* centerfolds and Miss America pageants weigh less than they did in the 1970s. In one analysis, 29 percent of recent *Playboy* centerfolds and 17 percent of Miss America pageant winners had BMIs below 17.5, the standard for being underweight.

In a study of college students, women failed to see themselves as underweight, even when they were, and perceived themselves as overweight, even when they were not. Many of the women who considered themselves normal weight nonetheless desired to be thinner.

You may think that you'll feel differently about your body and like it more when you weigh less. But whatever your weight or shape, you can improve your body esteem. How?

• Start walking with more bounce in your step.

• Focus on the parts of your body you like. Take pride in your beautiful eyes or graceful hands.

• Treat yourself with the respect you'd like to receive from others. Don't put yourself down or joke about your weight.

• Don't put off special plans, such as learning to kayak or taking a road trip to a national park, until you reach a certain magical weight: Do what you want to do *now*.

• Answer the following questions to remind yourself of why your body deserves love and appreciation.

> *Do your feet take you where you want to go?*
> *Does your tongue allow you to talk with your friends?*
> *Do your eyes allow you to see the people you love?*
> *Do your ears allow you to hear laughter and music?*
> *Do all your senses fill your life with beauty and wonder?*

On your way to a fitter body, enjoy the pleasures of the one you have.

55

How Are You Doing?

Yyou can't know how far you've come—or how far you have to go—unless you monitor your progress. Here are our suggestions for staying on top of your weight loss.

• **A quarter-day review.** Most dieters talk about good days and bad days. Rather than look at entire days as successes or failures, divide your waking hours into quarters and separately evaluate the morning quarter, the afternoon quarter, the early-evening quarter, and the late-evening quarter. When you think in these terms, it is hard for a day to be a complete bust. Even if you sneak a late-evening snack, you can still congratulate yourself for healthy eating in the other three quarters of the day, which will help keep up your morale.

• **A weekly weigh-in.** Weigh yourself at least once every week as a way of staying informed. Accept the number on your scale as simply a number, and don't attach feelings to it. Record your weight in your notebook, and next week weigh yourself and record your weight again. Continue to monitor your weight every week. View plateaus or occasional gains as temporary setbacks. By sticking with your weight-loss plan, in time you'll see the numbers decreasing.

• **A monthly measurement.** With a tape measure, check the size of your bust, waist, hips, thighs, and upper arms. A few weeks after you've started eating less and exercising more, check them again. This can help quantify the effects of working out. Even if you haven't lost weight, your body may be changing as you tone and strengthen your muscles.

• **A quarterly report card.** Play teacher, and make out your own report card. Get your journal and give yourself an A, B, C, D, or F for each of the following:

> *Has breakfast every day* ____
> *Eats nutritionally balanced meals* ____
> *Is physically active an hour or more each day* ____
> *Is conscious of and restricts sugar intake* ____
> *Understands the difference among carbohydrates, fat grams, protein, and calories* ____
> *Regularly uses a stress-management technique, such as meditation or an affirmation* ____
> *Doesn't overeat* ____
> *Limits saturated fats* ____
> *Rarely drinks more than one alcoholic beverage per day* ____
> *Takes recommended vitamins* ____
> *Checks weight once a week* ____
> *Drinks at least eight glasses of water a day* ____
> *Makes time for a personal pleasure every day* ____

If you have all As and Bs, you made the honor roll. Congratulations!

56

Mind Maps

People can get trapped in their own particular view of the world. Called belief systems by experts in neurolinguistic programming (NLP), these inner maps in your brain shape, empower, or limit your ability to reach your goals. If you believe in something—good or bad, fact or fiction—you act as if it were true. If you believe you can't stay on a diet, lose weight, or find time to exercise, you are setting yourself up for failure.

To open your eyes and challenge distorted beliefs, make a list of dietary actions that you think you cannot do. For example, "I can't give up bread and butter," "I can't stop eating sweets," or "I can't stop drinking soda."

In your notebook, rewrite the list and replace the words "I can't" with "I won't": "I won't give up bread and butter," "I won't stop eating sweets," or "I won't stop drinking soda." Saying, "I won't" affirms that *you* are in charge. As this realization takes root, you soon will be saying, "I can give up sweets."

To reinforce your new vision, stand in front of a mirror and tell yourself, "I *can* stay on my diet," "I *can* lose weight," "I *can* control my eating," "I *can* make time for 15 minutes of sit-ups and push-ups."

Changing the way you express yourself is a step toward changing your belief systems.

57

Are You Disinhibited?

Accoring to researchers at Tufts University, most thin people have low disinhibition levels. If they aren't hungry, no matter what mouth-watering delicacy they're offered, they just don't eat it. Heavier people have high disinhibition levels. No matter how full they feel, if offered something appealing, they eat it.

If you have high disinhibition, take heart. You can lower your disinhibition level over time so you won't be so tempted to eat regardless of whether or not you're hungry. Here are some ways to begin:

• Count calories conscientiously so you get used to eating normally as opposed to stuffing yourself.

• Limit the number of courses and dishes. When you are presented with too many options, you're much more likely to overeat because you'll want to try everything.

• Eat slowly and stop as soon as you begin to feel slightly full.

• Watch portion sizes. At restaurants, order a half portion or an appetizer as your dinner. Use the chart on page 138 when you're cooking or eating at home. Here are some easy ways to estimate appropriate serving sizes.

"Right Size" Your Servings

- A medium apple, orange, or cup of fruit = a baseball
- Half a cup of ice cream = a racquetball
- Three ounces of meat = a medium bar of soap
- A medium potato = a computer mouse
- An average bagel = a hockey puck
- Three ounces of grilled fish = a checkbook
- One ounce of cheese = four dice
- Two tablespoons of peanut butter = a golf ball
- Four small cookies = 4 poker chips
- A pancake = a CD

For the next month, write down each time you eat so much you feel that "you could pop." Then determine what caused your downfall—too many calories, too many choices, portions too large, eating too fast. Once you get a handle on why and how you stuff yourself, you'll be in a better position to take control of the amount of food you eat.

58
The Dog Ate My Diet

Children come up with all sorts of excuses to explain why they didn't do their homework. So do people trying to assure themselves that it's okay to overeat. Do any of these sound familiar?

Health excuses

- I haven't had any calcium today, so I'd better order a milk shake.
- My stomach hurts. I'd probably feel better if I had something to eat.

Giving-up excuses

- I'll never be thin anyway.
- I've worked hard today. I need nourishment.

Blaming excuses

- My husband doesn't like it when I watch my weight because we can't go to his favorite restaurants.
- My family likes me just the way I am.

Bedtime excuses

- I sleep better on a full stomach.
- I don't want to wake up hungry.

Celebration excuses

- It's my birthday.
- It's the day before my birthday.
- It's my best friend's birthday.
- It's Friday!

Victim excuses

- I'm the only one in my family who has to watch what she eats.
- I have a slow metabolism.

Your favorite excuses

What are your favorite excuses? Jot them in your weight-loss journal. The more aware you are of what you tell yourself when you want to overeat, the less likely you are to play the excuse game.

59

What's Your YLL?

Most people think of weight in terms of the excess pounds they need to lose but never think about what else they could lose if they don't lose weight: years of life.

Scientists have calculated the YLL—years of life lost—caused by obesity for individuals of different ages and weights. The younger you are, the more years of potential life you have to lose. If you are obese at age twenty-five, you stand to lose 8 years—13 percent of your projected life span. If you're forty, excess weight can trim 3.3 years from your life expectancy. For women, obesity increases the relative risk of dying by 50 percent compared to their thinner peers.

Consider what you might miss if your life were cut short: watching children grow, cherishing time with loved ones, spring blossoms, Thanksgiving get-togethers, summer vacations, birthdays, anniversaries, countless places you might have visited, laughs you might have shared, contributions you might have made.

Excess weight doesn't just slice years from the end of your life; it diminishes the quality of your life every day. The effects of obesity on health are the equivalent of twenty years of aging. Although your chronological age may be twenty-five, if you're obese, you're living in a middle-aged body. If you're forty-five, your body is getting ready for retirement. If you're sixty-five, your body is pushing its mortal limits.

As you work toward your goal of a leaner, healthier body, remind yourself that with every pound you lose you buy yourself a better and longer life.

60

Become an Advice Columnist

When you listen to others describe their weight problems, you may readily see what they should or shouldn't do. It's far more difficult to "step back," as neurolinguists put it, and view your own weight from a broader perspective. This exercise can help:

"Abby" for a day

If you ever wanted Dear Abby's job, here's your chance. Write your answers to the following questions from people with weight problems in your "Think Thin, Be Thin" notebook or computer file.

> Dear Abby,
>
> I believe a lot of my weight problem comes from where I work. We have a small lunch area on our floor, and people constantly bring birthday cakes, Danish pastries, and homemade cookies. No matter how much I tell myself I don't have to eat it, by 2:00 p.m. I've had some of everything.
>
> Do you have any suggestions?
>
> Signed,
Working in an Office
of Fatties

Dear Abby,

I come from an Italian background, and each Sunday a dozen of us—my parents, two sisters and a brother, and all of our families—get together at my parents' home. Mom's a wonderful cook, and a typical Sunday dinner usually includes two pastas, a main course, and homemade tiramisu for dessert. I don't want to hurt her feelings, but it's impossible not to overeat. Should I just stay home?

Signed,

A Dutiful Daughter

Dear Abby,

I feel so bad about myself. I can't seem to stop gaining weight. A year ago I lost forty pounds and was sooo happy. I got new clothes and felt like an entirely different woman. Today I've regained thirty of those pounds I fought so hard to lose. None of my friends have said much about the weight I've put back on, but I can imagine what they are thinking. Please, please, please help me.

Signed,

Missing Willpower

Although there is no one right answer to these letters, you probably came up with several useful suggestions. Because the problems weren't yours, you automatically stepped back from them and saw solutions.

Write "Dear Abby."

Now write to ask Dear Abby's help with a specific weight problem you face, such as overeating with friends or Saturday-night eating binges. After you describe the problem, play "Dear Abby" again, and write an answer.

The very act of writing allows you to step back, which empowers you to become more self-aware and self-accepting. You see more alternatives and gain flexibility—attributes that will serve you well for both losing weight and keeping it off.

61
Shape Your Way to Weight Loss

Shaping, a behavioral modification technique that uses rewards and incentives to motivate change, can reinforce your progress on the way to your shape-up goal.

Start by developing a list of positive reinforcements you'd like to give yourself. (See page 147.) Some can be pleasant experiences. Others might be gifts you purchase in advance and save for when you reach a goal. If that's too much of a test of your willpower, place items in an online shopping cart, and order only when you've earned a reward.

Using the techniques described in Tip 5, set a goal that is both a reach and reachable—for instance, engaging in ten minutes more of a physical activity three times a week. When you meet the goal, reward yourself. Think of it as giving yourself a gold star for a job well done. After a few weeks, add another ten minutes and an extra day to your goal before you earn a reward.

Over time continue to extend the time or effort needed to earn a reward. You might increase the number of days you work out during the week or the number of minutes of activity per day before you can claim a reward. After several months, most people find that they no longer need any tangible reinforcements. The pride they feel in taking better care of their bodies becomes incentive and reward enough.

Positive Reinforcers

A long walk

Sitting on a park bench and watching the ducks

Reading uninterrupted for twenty minutes

Listening to your favorite music

Looking through an old photo album

A bubble bath

A new pair of dazzling earrings

A temporary rinse in your hair

Calling a friend you haven't talked with in ages

Fresh flowers

A new fragrance

A makeover at a local department store

Getting yourself a pedicure

Watching a favorite classic movie

Sleeping in on Sunday

Make a list in your notebook of ten more rewards you might turn to instead of food.

62

The Hungry Brain

Your stomach may growl when empty, but hunger— the physiological drive to consume food—begins in the brain. Researchers at the National Institutes of Health have identified appetite receptors within the hypothalamus region of the brain that specifically respond to hunger messages carried by chemicals. In turn, hunger activates parts of the brain involved with emotions, thinking, and feeling.

Appetite, which is the psychological desire to eat, is a response to hunger. To avoid the unpleasant sensations of being hungry, we learn to eat a certain amount of food at certain times of the day, just as animals in the laboratory learn to avoid electric shocks by jumping at the sound of a warning bell.

Satiety is the feeling of fullness and relief from hunger that we feel by eating. The neurotransmitter serotonin has been shown to produce feelings of fullness. In addition, several peptides, released from the digestive tract as we ingest food, may signal the brain to stop or restrict eating. However, it takes twenty minutes for the brain to register fullness.

That's why you want to think of your hungry brain as

well as your hungry belly and stretch your meal times. To do so, try the following tactics:

• **Pause between bites.** At some point in your meal, pause—first for 30 seconds, then for longer periods. If you want second helpings, wait. If you find it hard to slow yourself down, choose foods that take time (and effort) to eat, such as artichokes, crab claws, and corn on the cob.

• **Try empty-handed eating.** Watch your hands at your next meal. Are you always holding something—knife, spoon, fork, dinner roll, glass of wine? If so, practice a new skill: emptying your hands after every bite. Initially, try not to pick up your fork for five seconds between bites. After a few meals, stretch the pause to ten, then fifteen seconds.

• **Switch hands.** For one meal each day, eat with your nondominant hand. It may feel awkward to switch your fork to your left or right hand, but opposite-hand eating forces you to focus on what you're putting on your fork and in your mouth.

• **Use chopsticks.** Eating with chopsticks—unless you're adept—also turns on your brain and slows down the pace of your meal. Try eating popcorn with chopsticks. You'll find that you can't shove five or six kernels into your mouth at a time as you usually would.

63

Self-Hypnosis

Once dismissed as the stuff of corny nightclub acts, hypnosis has won acceptance as a highly effective treatment for mental and physical problems. Named for Hypnos, the winged Greek god of sleep, hypnosis is a state of intense concentration that alters the way the brain accepts information. In a hypnotic trance, individuals focus so intently that they are unaware of sounds, sights, sensations (including pain), and other occurrences. In experimental studies, neuroscientists have documented clear changes in the electrical activity of the brains of hypnotized subjects.

Hynosis in itself is not a form of therapy, but it can be used in therapeutic ways. Because of their intense concentration, sometimes referred to as their "altered state of consciousness," hypnotized subjects are more accepting of instructions and "posthypnotic suggestions" designed to influence behavior after the session is over.

Hypnosis does not take away will; instead it suspends the tendency to challenge or criticize. This is why it's particularly effective in breaking bad habits, such as smoking and overeating. Most people are excellent candidates for hypnosis. With know-how and practice, you can learn to hypnotize yourself and attain the same benefits you would with a therapist.

Although you may not realize it, you experience a trance-like state when you daydream or become so engrossed that you don't hear someone talking to you. When you hypnotize yourself, you do the same thing: you relax, block out most stimuli, focus, and give yourself suggestions. You might tell yourself, "I eat slowly and only when hungry," or "The first thing I do in the morning is walk on my treadmill." Your unconscious mind stores the messages like other data. The messages then come back to you when you sit down to eat or wake in the morning.

Learning to block out stimuli and become deeply relaxed takes practice, just like anything else. We suggest that you hypnotize yourself twice a day the first week, once a day the second week, and then every three or four days. A self-hypnosis session takes only ten to fifteen minutes.

Ready to try?

Go to a room where you won't be interrupted. Decide on the hypnotic suggestion you plan to give yourself. Write it down, and then memorize it. Get comfortable, take off your shoes, and relax. Breathe deeply and rhythmically, slowly taking the air in and slowly letting it out. As you're breathing, stare at something in the room, such as a lamp or paperweight. Tell yourself you're feeling very relaxed. Then close your eyes and focus on breathing and relaxing.

Begin counting, starting with the number one and continuing up to thirty. As you count, focus on your breathing. Relax your head; relax your neck; relax your shoulders, arms, hands, legs, and feet. Allow yourself to drift and become totally relaxed.

When you reach thirty, give yourself the hypnotic suggestion you've memorized—for example, "Fresh fruits and vegetables are my favorite snack food." Repeat your suggestion several times while continuing to focus on your breathing. Then count from thirty back to number one. As you count backward, you'll become more aware of your surroundings. When you reach the number one, say aloud, "You did a good job." Open your eyes, look around, and reorient yourself.

It may take four or five tries to feel yourself slipping into a hypnotic trance, but don't give up. If you're still having a particularly hard time, seek the help of a therapist who uses hypnosis regularly and can teach you self-hypnosis in one session.

64

Give Thanks

According to researchers in the field of positive psychology, which studies the healthy and helpful aspects of human nature, a grateful spirit brightens mood, boosts energy, and infuses daily living with a sense of glad abundance. Because it reminds them that life has been good to them in the past, gratitude may protect people from emotional eating and make them more aware of what and why they eat. In psychological studies, people who felt thankful for life's blessings were more likely to be fit.

You can consciously become more grateful by registering the good things happening in your life. Asked to record things they're grateful for every day, volunteers in psychological experiments reported more positive feelings, more energy, and better sleep. They felt richer, regardless of how much money they had. And the full of heart may not need to keep their stomachs so full.

How can you help your gratitude grow? Here are some suggestions:

• In your notebook, make a list of the blessings in your life. Start with whatever you're most grateful for—family, home, job—and keep looking for what else is going right in your life: a new puppy, a soft bed with sweet-smelling sheets, a drawing your child makes for you at school.

• Develop a "good" memory, one that stores the kindnesses and comforts that have come your way. Pay attention to the small acts of generosity and caring that happen every day, even gestures as small as someone letting you slip ahead of them in a cashier's line.

• Build thankfulness into your day. An ideal time is before a meal, with or without a traditional grace. Pausing to take a few breaths and reflect on your day not only soothes the soul but sets the stage for mindful eating.

65

Break the See-Food, Eat-Food Syndrome

Some people are especially "disinhibited" (see Tip 57) or susceptible to cues that trigger eating. They eat when others eat, when they see commercials for food, or when they spot a soft-pretzel vendor. We call this the see-food, eat-food syndrome. If you eat in response to environmental cues, develop "skillpower" rather than trying to rely solely on willpower. The following suggestions can help:

• **Avoid temptation.** Rid your shelves of calorie-laden foods you don't love but eat just because they're there. Remove dishes of candies or nuts from the house. Store high-fat foods in the back of the freezer or pantry. At mealtime, leave serving dishes in the kitchen and eat in the dining room so you aren't looking at food and have to think twice before taking seconds. Don't go to the dry cleaner located next to the ice-cream shop, or rest in a chair near the food court at the mall.

• **Stay away from crowds.** If you limit your number of dinner companions, you'll also limit how much you eat. According to researchers, the more individuals at your table, the more you'll eat, regardless of whether you're hungry.

When you eat with a group or your family, don't feel

you need to eat everything they eat. See if you can eat more slowly or less than they do.

• **"This Little Piggy . . ."** If you usually raid the refrigerator at night, put a bell on the door or a fluorescent sticker that says, "Stop." A woman we know has a little plastic pig in her refrigerator. When the door opens and the refrigerator light goes on, the little pig squeals, "Oink, oink, oink, oink." Does the little piggy halt a planned food fest? Sometimes yes, sometimes no. But it always increases awareness. Can you think of something you might do to increase your awareness as you swing open the refrigerator door? What about a picture of the body you'd like to have with your head pasted over the model's? Or a yellow ribbon tied around the handle to signify *Caution*.

66

Dresses for Diet Success

What are you wearing right now?

A belt—or pants with an elastic waistband? A buttoned blouse—or an oversized sweatshirt? As they put on weight, many women try to hide under shapeless, bulky clothes. We suggest you come out from under, do a reality check, and wear clothes that make you more body conscious.

Think of your wardrobe as a form of biofeedback. Wear pants or a skirt that zips. Keep your belt snug to remind you to sit and stand straighter, suck in your stomach, and skip the second helpings. If you're self-conscious about a flabby waist, wear your shirt over your slacks. In time you'll prefer it tucked.

Pay attention to the way you feel as you button your blouse or squeeze into jeans. Do they tug or pinch when you bend or sit? Do they feel tighter after lunch? Catch your reflection in a window or mirror. Imagine a day when the outfit you're wearing will feel baggy.

When heading for an occasion of potential overeating, choose what you wear with your weight in mind. If you put on your "skinny" slacks, they'll remind you to hold back at the buffet.

Use clothes to maintain motivation as you diet. In spring, as you count down to swimsuit season, hang a bathing suit somewhere you can't help but notice—next to your mirror, perhaps. Excavate the tight skirt you haven't fit into for years from the back of your closet, and keep it in plain sight.

As you lose weight, don't hang on to your "fat" clothes in case you need them again. You won't. Give them away to a shelter or charity.

67

How Were You "Scripted"?

Regardless of their training and approach, therapists always ask about a patient's childhood because they are looking for clues to how the person was "scripted," that is, overtly and covertly instructed in living. Although you may not be aware of it, your childhood scripting about food and eating may play a role in your weight problem.

If you were forced to eat everything on your plate, for instance, you may believe that you should eat what's in front of you, regardless of how full you feel. If dessert was always a part of dinner, you may feel deprived if you don't have something sweet to finish a meal.

In order to become more aware of how early-childhood lessons affect your eating habits and weight, answer the following questions in your "Think Thin, Be Thin" notebook. The more fully you answer them, the more insight you will acquire. Once you can see your answers in writing, you'll be better able to decide whether to change or continue to follow your childhood script.

I. How were meals handled in your family? Did Mom do the cooking and Dad the grilling? Did you sit down to dinner at a certain time? Or did your family eat in fast-food restaurants or in the car in between dance classes and music lessons?

2. Were there any rituals before or during dinner, such as your parents' having a cocktail or the family saying grace out loud?

3. Did the entire family eat together, or did people eat individually? Was the atmosphere at mealtime tense or relaxed, enjoyable or strained? Did you talk, laugh, sit in silence, argue, watch television?

4. Was snacking between meals allowed and what types of snacks were you permitted to eat and drink? Candy bars? Cookies? Fruit? Chips? Crackers? Soda? Milk? Juice?

5. What were you taught, directly or indirectly, about what to eat and drink, how to eat, how much to eat, how fast or slow to eat?

6. Was a parent's weight or your weight an issue when you were a child?

7. Did you feel you were too thin, too fat, or just the right size? How did you get this idea?

8. Did anything happen in childhood regarding your weight and eating that has significantly affected your life today? What was it?

9. What do you wish your parents had done differently regarding meals and snacks?

10. What do you wish they had said to you about your eating, your body, or your weight?

Review your answers. Is anything in your childhood script getting in the way of your losing weight? If so, do what Hollywood scriptwriters do: Rewrite it.

68

How Do You Blow Your Diet?

As you read these seven common ways of falling off the weight-loss wagon, mentally check off those that apply to you:

_____ I. Once I overeat, I keep stuffing myself the rest of the day.

_____ 2. I don't keep track of what I eat.

_____ 3. I don't weigh myself.

_____ 4. I can't resist cravings.

_____ 5. I reach for food when stressed.

_____ 6. If the scale shows that I've gained a pound, I console myself with food.

_____ 7. I tell myself that today I can eat what I want because tomorrow I'll go back on a diet.

Which of the actions you checked has contributed the most to your weight gain?

Read through the following list and mentally check the changes you're willing to make.

_____ I. If I find that I'm stuffing myself, I will take a sip of water or put a piece of gum in my mouth and tell myself, "It's over."

_____ 2. I will record everything I eat for the next three days.

_____ 3. I will weigh myself every week.

_____ 4. I will wait ten minutes before giving in to a craving.

_____ 5. I will spend time every day calming my mind through meditation, progressive relaxation, or saying my affirmation.

_____ 6. I will refuse to let a number on a scale derail my diet.

_____ 7. I will tell myself that I choose to watch what I eat today.

Write the changes you intend to make in your "Think Thin, Be Thin" notebook.

69
Stress-Proofing

You know about stress. You live with it every day: deadlines on a major project at work, credit-card debt, a car crash, a leaking roof. As researchers have demonstrated, the day-in, day-out stressors of modern life keep levels of hormones like cortisol elevated. One way to lower them is to stimulate the pleasure centers in the brain. The most popular way of doing this? Eating, particularly foods high in fat and sugar such as chocolate bars and ice cream.

Even a temporary stressor, such as speaking in public, affects food choices. In one experiment, British researchers divided sixty-eight men and women into two groups: Half were told to prepare a four-minute speech, which would be filmed and evaluated after lunch. The scientists told the other half that they would listen to a reading after lunch. Both groups served themselves from a buffet that included sweet, salty, bland, high-fat, and low-fat foods. Those anticipating the stress of public speaking did not report larger appetites or eat more food, but they ate more sweet, high-fat foods, which have a calming effect on brain chemistry.

Although you can't avoid stress, you can keep it from

sidetracking your diet and exercise plan. Here are some strategies that can help:

• Watch for warning signals of stress overload, such as problems sleeping or concentrating, irritability, headaches, or becoming accident-prone.

• Master a relaxation technique, such as meditation, visualization, progressive relaxation, or mindful breathing. (See Tips 45, 90, 38, 30.) Practice your relaxation technique instead of trying to munch away stress.

• Because physical activity both lowers stress and helps you lose weight, make time to exercise every day. If you don't have an hour to work out, make it thirty minutes. If you don't have thirty, go for fifteen. Maintaining the routine of a daily workout will keep you on track and motivated for when you have a little more time to spare.

• If you have to travel, before you leave home make a plan for remaining active. Find out if your hotel has a fitness center or gym. Check on nearby walking paths. Bring your bathing suit if there's a pool.

• If you know you'll be working late, stock a desk drawer with small boxes of raisins, packages of dried soup, and other low-calorie snacks. If you'll be eating out, decide what types of food—a healthy salad and fish entrée, for instance—you'll order and which ones you'll avoid. If you'll be in the company of hearty eaters, practice eating more slowly than anyone at the table.

• If you're so stressed out that you're tempted to soothe yourself with food, release the tension by getting physical. Pretend you're a boxer, and throw punches into the air. Try some karate kicks forward, backward, and to each side. Grunting while boxing or kicking the air intensifies the feeling of relief. If you need a quick and convenient tension buster, try the stress press described below.

Stress Press

- Either stand up or lean forward in your chair.
- Press the palms of your hands together and rub furiously, getting your forearms and elbows moving.
- Bend over more. Press your palms together even more tightly and keep rubbing. Continue for two or three minutes.

You should feel a lot less tense—and less likely to crave a snack. This works because the vigorous rubbing diverts blood flow from your stomach to your hands. Switching focus to the exercise also gives your mind a break.

70

Is More Better?

If you began exercising as part of your weight-loss program, bravo! Maybe you're walking a mile longer, jogging a full minute faster, or hoisting eight-pound weights for biceps curls. How much farther, faster, or harder do you have to work?

We don't blame you if you aren't sure. Various health organizations have endorsed different minimums. The Centers for Disease Control and Prevention and the American College of Sports Medicine recommend thirty minutes a day of moderate activity. But the Institute of Medicine suggests sixty minutes of moderate exercise as the minimum needed to maintain a healthy weight.

How much exercise really is enough? The answer may surprise you.

In one recent study, 184 sedentary, overweight women between ages 21 and 45 all cut back their food intake to between 1,200 and 1,500 calories a day and walked at varying intensities from 30 to 60 minutes a day 5 days a week. Researchers expected that more effort would bring greater benefits. It did, but the difference was minimal.

Women who walked for thirty minutes a day lost an average of fourteen pounds over a year. Those who worked out vigorously for an hour a day lost twenty pounds. All the women also improved their cardiovascular fitness and lowered their breast-cancer risk—whether they exercised moderately or vigorously.

What mattered more than exertion, the researchers concluded, was commitment. Of the women who stayed with the program for a year—as more than 94 percent did—all lost at least 10 percent of their weight. Slow and steady may not win the race, but it can peel away pounds and keep them off.

71

Stop the Yo-Yo

Although diets do take off pounds, if you view them as an aberration from everyday life, you'll eventually go back to your old eating habits and regain the weight you lost.

If you've been losing (and regaining) the same five or ten pounds for years, try the following suggestions for long-term success:

• **Don't go to extremes.** On-and-off dieting, especially by means of very-low-calorie diets (under 800 calories a day), can be self-defeating and dangerous. Weight that goes down too fast inevitably comes back up, often higher than before. Repeated cycles of rapid weight loss followed by weight gain can take a toll on health and may even change food preferences. Chronic crash dieters often come to prefer high-calorie, low-nutrition foods that combine sugar and fat, such as cake frosting.

• **Set a danger zone.** Once you've reached your desired weight, don't let your weight climb more than three or four pounds higher. Take into account normal fluctuations, but watch out for an upward trend. Once you hit your upper weight limit, take action immediately rather than waiting until you gain ten pounds.

• **Stay active.** Researchers at the University of Pennsylvania found that when women who exercised shifted to the maintenance stage of their diet, their metabolism remained the same. On the other hand, the metabolism of women who dieted without exercising slowed, and when they stopped dieting, they started gaining weight.

• **Be patient.** Think of weight loss like a road trip. If you're going across town, you expect to get there in twenty minutes. If your destination is four hundred miles away, you know it'll take longer. Give yourself the time you need to lose weight safely and steadily.

• **Try, try again.** Dieters don't usually keep weight off on their first attempt. The people who eventually succeed don't give up. Through trial and error they find a plan that works for them.

72

Putting Your Dreams to Work

We all dream three to five times a night. Although scientists have never been able to explain why, dreams seem critical to processing life events. Some dreams appear to reflect daily life, while others may provide insight into a difficult problem. Bad dreams sometimes feel like warnings, alerting you to something you may be avoiding or denying.

If you're struggling with your weight, tell yourself right before falling to sleep, "Tonight I'll have a dream, and in my dream I'll find help with my weight." If you don't succeed the first night, give yourself the same message the following night. With repeated effort, most people can remember their dreams and often find the help they wanted. Another option to help you recall a dream is to set your alarm for ten to fifteen minutes earlier so you're more likely to catch yourself dreaming.

The next time you remember a dream, try analyzing it. This example from one of the women in our weight-loss group can show you how.

Katie dreamed she was pushing a wheelbarrow up a steep hill strewn with large reddish rocks. As she pushed, she noticed beautiful larkspur along the road and felt while looking at the flowers a sense of peace. However, her overall feeling was fear that she wasn't strong enough to make it to the top of the hill.

We told Katie to pick out three items in her dream. She chose the wheelbarrow, the rocks, and the larkspur. Drawing on Gestalt therapy, which views dreams as projections or statements about the dreamer's life, we asked her to become each object she had chosen by using the pronoun I. This technique helps the dreamer identify more closely with the object.

Here is what Katie found:

"I am a wheelbarrow. I'm made of heavy metal, and I work hard. I'm determined to get myself up the hill. It may take awhile, but I'll get there if my wheels hold out."

"I am the rocks in the road, and I'm here to make the job of pushing the wheelbarrow up the hill even harder. Maybe I'll even be able to stop the wheelbarrow from getting to the top of the hill."

"I am the lavender larkspur on the side of the hill. I'm strong, and I've pushed my way up through this rocky terrain. I give beauty to the passersby. People take strength from seeing me."

After this exercise, Katie said she could see that losing weight was an uphill battle, just like pushing the wheelbarrow up the hill. But despite the many obstacles—she equated the rocks in the road with all the snacks at her office and social events, which often centered around food—she felt she could lose the weight she wanted to lose. Katie decided to keep a purple flower on her table as a reminder that she too was strong like the purple flowers that had found their way through the rock—strong enough to reach her weight-loss goal.

Is this what Katie's dream really meant? No one can say, but Katie's interpretation of her dream helped her lose weight.

Another approach to dream analysis, also rooted in Gestalt therapy, is to write down a dream. In your notebook make a list of every person, place, thing, and feeling you can remember from your dream. Let's say that your list includes your grandmother, a beautiful blue parrot, a cup of tea, and a feeling of sadness.

After making your list, we would ask you to close your eyes, and ask your grandmother why she's in your dream. You would ask the same question of the beautiful blue parrot, the cup of tea, and the feeling of sadness. Then go further with your analysis, and ask yourself:

- Was I avoiding anything in my dream?
- Was I trying to escape or hide from something?
- How is my dream similar to the issues I'm struggling with in my waking hours?
- Is my dream sending me a message?

This dream exercise can help both in starting and in keeping you on the road to weight loss. If you belong to a weight-loss group, take turns sharing what each of you has discovered in your dreams.

73

Tease Your Mind

Parables, one of the oldest forms of instruction, move the mind away from habitual ways of thinking and get a person to look at life from a different perspective. Therapists trained in neurolinguistic programming (NLP) understand that a parable can be as effective as several therapy sessions in helping a client achieve his or her goals.

We think the following parable may give you the added insight and help you need to achieve your weight-loss goal. Read over the following paraphrased parable from *The Miracle of Change*, by Dennis Wholey.

A man is swimming across a river. In one hand he holds a big rock. As he nears the middle of the river, the people on the shore can see that the man is in trouble. He's choking and sputtering. He's struggling to stay afloat.

"Drop the rock!" one man shouts. "You'll be able to swim better."

But the man in the water clings to the rock. Everyone on shore realizes that he is drowning.

"Drop the rock!" the people shout. "Drop the rock!"

Finally the man turns. With his last breath he gasps, "I can't. It's mine."

Now take out your "Think Thin, Be Thin" notebook or open your computer file and answer the following questions.

Thinking of your weight as the rock:

• Do you see your weight as pulling you down?
• Do you see yourself holding on to your weight despite impending disaster?
• Are there others in your life, like the people on shore, trying to encourage you to lose weight?

The man justifies his behavior by saying that the rock is his and therefore he can't let go of it. How do you justify your weight?

Is there anything anyone could say or do to convince you to let go of your weight?

If you are in a weight-loss group, use this exercise to launch a discussion.

74

Dangerous Thinking

- "I've worked all week. I've earned a night off my diet."
- "Every woman in our family is fat. Why should I expect to be thin?"
- "I get enough exercise chasing my two kids around the house."

Psychologists refer to statements like these as "facilitating thoughts," rationalizations that allow us not to do what we know we should.

Are your thoughts sabotaging your weight loss? For a day or two, tune in to what's going through your mind as you take a second scoop of mashed potatoes or skip your "butts and guts" exercise class. Jot down these thoughts in your "Think Thin, Be Thin" notebook or computer file. Once you raise your awareness of facilitating thoughts, launch a counterattack. Several times a day tell yourself, "I'll eat only when I'm hungry." Before you put anything in your mouth, pause, and ask a single question: "Am I really hungry?" If not, just don't eat it.

Do the same with exercise. Remind yourself periodically, "Exercise is my top priority." When thoughts about errands to run threaten to short-circuit your workout, ask yourself, "What's my top priority?" Then lace up your shoes and just do it.

75

Why Good Diets Go Bad

You've heard the gloomy words before: Diets don't work. People who lose weight always regain it. Fat is forever.

Don't believe the doomsayers. You can lose weight and keep it off. In surveys of people who lost significant amounts of weight and kept it off for several years, most did so on their own—without medication, meal substitutes, or membership in an organized weight-loss group. When a National Institutes of Health panel reviewed forty-eight separate weight-loss trials, they found that participants lost about 8 percent of their body weight on average and kept it off.

If your diet is no longer working for you, however, do some detective work. Here are some questions to ask:

• **Are you eating too little?** If you restrict yourself to fewer than 800 to 1,000 calories a day, you are, in effect, starving. Your body responds by using less and less energy. Your metabolic rate goes down by as much as 20 to 25 percent; your pulse slows; your body starts breaking down muscle tissue. Sooner or later, "restricted" eaters, as they're sometimes called, can deny themselves no more. They succumb to a craving, often end up bingeing—and blow their diet.

• **Do you rely on prepared diet products?** While you'll lose weight on prepackaged diet drinks and foods, you eventually have to face the real-food challenge. When you do, you may feel an uncontrollable urge to overeat. Low- and no-fat foods can also boomerang. In recent studies, individuals who used artificial sweeteners or drank only diet drinks were more likely to gain weight than those who didn't. The reason: Many people feel so virtuous about giving up fat or sugar that they think they've "earned" a second helping or high-calorie treat.

• **Is your diet too bland?** Low-calorie foods like nonfat cottage cheese or yogurt can make you yearn for more interesting tastes and textures. If you're giving up rich foods, try highly spiced dishes. A Virgin Mary makes a satisfying aperitif. If you choose a hot Indian curry as a main course, you'll be less likely to yearn for dessert. Dishes made with tongue-tingling chili peppers not only deliver more flavor bang for your caloric buck, but can help you burn off extra pounds by stoking up post-meal metabolism.

• **Are you too tough on yourself?** If you diet too zealously, you'll only set yourself up for failure. Rather than aiming for perfection, if you practice good eating habits 95 percent of the time a few indiscretions won't make a difference. Think in terms of choices, rather than imperatives.

• **Are you on a dubious diet?** The problem may not be you, but the weight-loss product or program you're using. The telltale signs of dangerous or fraudulent diets include promises of very rapid weight loss, claims that the diet can eliminate "cellulite" (the dimply fatty tissue on the thighs or buttocks), "counselors" who are really salespersons pushing a product or program, no mention of risks associated with the diet, and unproved gimmicks (such as body wraps, starch blockers, hormones, diuretics, or "unique" pills or potions). Another red flag: no maintenance program.

76

The Bottom Line

What has your weight cost you? In addition to the toll on mind and body, you literally pay a price for excess pounds, especially if you're a well-educated woman. In a recent study in Finland, obese women with white-collar jobs earned about 30 percent less—a difference of at least $5,000 a year—than normal-weight or even plump women. Weight had no significant impact on men's pay or on the pay of women who were poorly educated or manual workers.

Weight also may cost you a job or a promotion. In an unusual experiment, researchers videotaped mock job interviews in which professional actors appeared either as normal-weight or overweight applicants. When they wore makeup and prostheses that made them look thirty pounds heavier, the actors, using the same words, intonations, and gestures, were rated as less worthy of hiring. This bias occurred with both sexes but was especially strong against women applicants.

Unfair?

Absolutely. But weight discrimination occurs at every stage of the employment process: hiring, placement, and compensation. Can you fight it? Maybe. But you also can change your weight for your next job interview or salary review.

77

The Power of a Paradox

Just when you're on a weight-loss roll—eating right, working out, losing weight—you may suddenly revert back to your old unhealthy habits. You tell yourself to get back on the program, but somehow you can't—or won't.

Therapists refer to this phenomenon as "psychological reactance." When you perceive a threat to your "freedom" or feel that others are trying to limit your behavior, you unconsciously start to resist. Consciously you want to limit your eating and continue your exercise routine, but unconsciously, because you feel that you're losing your freedom, you become resistant.

How can you counteract these self-defeating responses?

One way is to give yourself a "paradoxical directive," a technique that is sometimes referred to as "prescribing the symptom." For example, suppose you just finished your second bowl of mocha-chip ice cream and are thinking about a third one. A good paradoxical directive would be to tell yourself, "Go ahead, have a third bowl. Gain another two pounds." By telling yourself this, you put yourself back in the driver's seat, feel free to make a choice, and no longer need to rebel against not being able to eat what you want.

If you follow the directive and eat the ice cream, you have nothing to lose since you were about to do so anyway. If you decide not to follow the directive, as often happens, you will find yourself back on the weight-loss track.

In the "double bind," you give yourself permission to make another bad choice. When you peer in the pantry or refrigerator for a snack, encourage yourself to eat everything in sight. Tell yourself it's okay to eat the entire tub of whipped cream cheese as well as the leftover bowl of spaghetti. Because you have given yourself permission to eat whatever you want, you feel back in control and can consciously decide to limit yourself. Do the same with exercise. Rather than haranguing yourself to go to the gym, give yourself permission to stay home and be a couch potato. At worse, you won't exercise. But if the paradoxical directive works—as it usually does—you'll be raring to work out.

Paradoxical directives are some of the most powerful tools therapists use when someone gets off track. However, we don't recommend them in the beginning of your weight-loss efforts. Do, however, put directives to work for you if you're at a weight-loss impasse. By breaking through the psychological reactance barrier, you can stop getting in your own way.

78
Go Unplugged

Atypical American woman watches thirty-four hours of television per week. Experts debate whether that much television is harmful to your brain, but it's definitely hazardous to your body. According to medical estimates, TV is a culprit in at least 30 percent of cases of obesity.

How does watching TV make you fat?

It takes up time you otherwise might spend doing something physical. Because people tend to snack while watching, they consume more food than they otherwise would. And compared with sewing, reading, driving, or other sedentary pursuits, watching TV lowers metabolic rate, so you burn fewer calories.

Even if you're not heavy, TV increases the odds that you will be. In a six-year study of almost 4,000 women who started out at normal weight, those who spent the most time watching television and the least time exercising ended up obese.

Do you have to pull the plug on your television? Not necessarily. But don't eat while watching. Find an activity like knitting, folding laundry, or ironing that may occupy your hands and keep up your metabolism as you watch.

Click the mute button during food commercials to avoid brainwashing. Better yet, do a few stretches or jog in place. And rethink how much time you really want to give to watching. When you watch instead of do, you become mentally and physically sluggish, which translates into boredom and weight gain.

79

Naikan

Naikan is a Japanese method of self-reflection that encourages one to "look inside." Gregg Krech, author of *Naikan*, explains that there are three simple questions that free you from focusing on *your* problems and shift your attention to feelings of appreciation *for others*. As this internal shift occurs, your troubles—including your struggle to lose weight—become less important for a time.

To try Naikan, think of a person close to you (mate, colleague, parent, sibling, teacher, or friend) and answer the following three questions:

1. What have I received from this person?
2. What have I given to this person?
3. What difficulties or troubles have I brought to this person?

Spend at least fifteen minutes on this exercise. We suggest you write your reflections in your "Think Thin, Be Thin" notebook or computer file. For the next several months, repeat this exercise each day, choosing a new person each time. This exercise provides a better understanding of your connection to others and an increased sense of behaving responsibly with others and within yourself. As your desire to act responsibly increases, you will find a spillover to all parts of your life. In its unique and gentle way, Naikan can renew your resolve to keep you moving toward a healthier weight.

80

One in Six

That's how many cancer deaths weight loss could prevent. A recent study of 900,000 people, the largest ever of its kind, found that excess weight may account for 14 to 20 percent of all cancer. Obesity has been implicated in cancers of the breast, uterus, cervix, ovary, stomach, prostate, colon and rectum, kidney, esophagus, pancreas, liver, and gallbladder, and in non-Hodgkin's lymphoma and multiple myeloma. Women who gain more than twenty pounds from age eighteen to midlife double their risk of breast cancer compared to women whose weight remains stable.

Too much body fat can increase cancer risk in several ways: It raises the amount of estrogen in the blood, which may contribute to cancers of the female reproductive system. It also raises levels of insulin, which prompts the body to create a hormone that causes cells to multiply. Acid reflux, which can cause cancer of the esophagus, occurs more frequently in heavy men and women. Obesity also makes various types of cancer harder to diagnose and treat.

Cancer is the disease most people fear most. You can fear less if you reduce your weight.

81

Secrets of Big Losers

Rather than focusing on why dieters fail, the creators of the National Weight Control Registry study the habits and lifestyles of those who've maintained a weight loss of at least 30 pounds for at least a year. The nearly 4,000 people in the registry have averaged a weight loss of 66 pounds, which they've kept off for 5.5 years.

No one diet or commercial weight-loss program helped all these formerly fat individuals. Many, through years of trial and error, eventually came up with a permanent exercise and eating program that worked for them. Despite the immense variety, their customized approaches share certain characteristics:

• **Personal responsibility for change.** Weight-loss winners develop an internal locus of control. (See Tip 11.) Rather than blaming others for their weight problem or relying on a doctor or trainer to fix it, they believe that the keys to a healthy weight lie within themselves.

• **Exercise.** Registry members report an hour of moderate physical activity almost every day. Their favorite exercise? Three in four say walking, followed by cycling, weightlifting, aerobics, running, and stair climbing. On average, they burn about 2,545 calories per week through physical activity.

• **Monitoring.** About 44 percent of the registry members count calories, and almost all keep track of their food intake in some way, written or not.

• **Vigilance.** Rather than avoiding the scale or telling themselves their jeans shrank in the wash, long-term losers keep tabs on their weight and size. About a third check the scale every week. If the scale notches upward or their waistband starts to pinch, they take action.

• **A low-fat diet.** Women in the registry who limited fat to 25 percent of daily calories kept off the greatest share of their lost weight. This is lower than the average 35 to 40 percent that most people eat, but well above the 10 percent or so recommended in low-fat diets.

• **Minimeals.** Registry members tend to eat between four and five meals or snacks every day. One meal most never missed: breakfast.

82

Breakfast Like a Champion

Your mother probably told you that breakfast is the most important meal of the day, and forty years of breakfast-related studies have proved her right. A morning meal improves concentration and problem-solving ability, boosts energy levels, and helps control weight. Regular breakfast skippers are four times more likely to be obese than those who eat a morning meal.

Breakfast does good for both body and mind. People who start the day with breakfast are less likely to crave a midmorning snack or to stuff themselves at lunch. They consume less overall fat during the day and have lower cholesterol levels than skippers. They also benefit psychologically. When you start your morning by eating something nutritious, you set yourself up for other healthy practices, like taking a walk and eating healthy foods, the rest of the day.

No time to whip up a hot breakfast? No problem. One of the best breakfasts is the simplest: ready-to-eat cereal or microwaveable oatmeal topped with berries or a banana. The soluble fiber in whole-grain cereals and oatmeal helps regulate metabolism and digestion, stabilize blood glucose, and lower the risk of heart disease. Because fiber slows the emptying of the stomach, you feel fuller and less hungry four to eight hours later. Another high-nutrition option is a smoothie (milk, fruit and a teaspoon of bran, whirled in a blender).

If you usually skip breakfast, it may take awhile to get used to this new pattern, because at first you won't have an appetite in the morning. But if you feed yourself first thing in the morning every day for three weeks, you'll start waking up hungry.

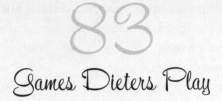

83
Games Dieters Play

This time Erin was sure she'd lose the extra weight she put on after breaking her leg two years ago. Then her husband, Matt, returned from a "doughnut run" with Erin's favorites as a treat. That was the end of her diet. "If it wasn't for Matt and those doughnuts," she tells everyone, "I'd still be on my diet."

Although neither realizes it, Matt and Erin are playing a "game," although not the recreational sort. In his groundbreaking book *Games People Play*, psychiatrist Eric Berne, the developer of transactional analysis, revealed the ways in which people engage in unhealthy, repetitive ways of interacting for the sake of gaining certain psychological advantages.

In this case, Matt may have bought the doughnuts because, on a unconscious basis, he doesn't want Erin to continue to lose weight. If she does lose her weight, he may have to deal with his overspending problem. Erin, on the other hand, may have been looking for an excuse to stop dieting. When Matt walked in the door with the doughnuts, she had her excuse.

The way out of this no-win game is for Erin to stop

blaming her husband and recognize that if she wants to stay on a diet, she can.

Have you ever played "If It Weren't for You"? Or do you play a variation, such as:

"If it weren't for my husband's cooking . . ."

"If it weren't for all the goodies everyone brings to work . . ."

"If it weren't for the family picnics . . ."

If you recognize playing this game, the first step is to admit it. Try to pinpoint the psychological payoff you are gaining. Then come up with specific strategies to end the game. Instead of blaming your husband's cooking, buy him a low-fat cookbook. Bring healthy snacks to work rather than munching on others' sweets. Take a platter of veggies to the next family gathering as an alternative to the potato salad.

"I'll Do It When I Get Damn Good and Ready"

After putting on twenty-five pounds in the last year, Lindsay asked her mother, Sally, for ten sessions with a personal trainer as a birthday present. Sally said sure and gave her a gift certificate for ten sessions. After several months, Sally asked if Lindsay had called the trainer. Lindsay said not yet. Two months later, Sally asked again. When Sally asked the third time about the trainer, Lindsay snapped, "I'll do it when I get damn good and ready."

By playing this game, Lindsay proved that nobody could tell her what to do. Instead of wasting her time engaged in such a fruitless power struggle, Lindsay would be well advised to schedule her first appointment with the trainer or to return the gift certificate and use the money to buy a treadmill.

"Why Don't You, Yes, But"

For years Emily has complained that no matter what she tries, she can't lose weight.

"Why don't you try Weight Watchers?" Jennifer, her best friend, asks.

"Yes, but I don't have time for weekly meetings," Emily replies.

"Why don't you skip the meetings and just follow the diet?" Jennifer suggests.

"Yes, but I hate the idea of having to count points," says Emily.

Jennifer tries another tack: "Why don't we join a gym together?"

Emily's response: "Yes, we could do that, but who would watch the kids?"

Emily and Jennifer are playing, "Why Don't You, Yes, But." This game allows Emily to talk about her concerns while avoiding doing anything about them. The game also puts Emily in control because nothing anyone says makes an impact.

In order to stop this game, Emily has to stop complaining about her weight and decide to do something about it, like following one of her friend's suggestions.

If you play games like these, figure out the unhealthy reasons why, and decide what you can do to stop playing and get serious about weight loss.

When You Hit a
Weight-Loss Wall

As they cut back on food and increase their activity, most dieters see their scales notch downward. But as metabolic rate adjusts to a lower calorie intake, calorie burning slows, and so does your weight loss. Even if you're doing everything right, you're bound to hit a weight plateau. For days—even weeks —the scale may not budge. The reason is that your body is readjusting its metabolic rate. To nudge the scale downward, try the following:

• Gather data. Go back to keeping a detailed food log for a week, including a weekend, and write down what you eat, when and where you eat it, what prompts your eating (emotions, hunger, etc.). You may find hidden calories.

• Reassess portion sizes. Even on high-protein diets, bigger portions mean more calories. Read food labels. Remember that low-fat doesn't mean low-calorie. Have you found some subtle ways of breaking your diet plan, such as an extra splash of milk in your coffee, a few more sprinkles of sugar in your tea, or another slice of meat in your sandwich? It may not feel like cheating, but when it comes to food, there are no harmless flirtations. So don't fool yourself into thinking these indulgences don't count. They do.

• Check with your doctor. Various medical conditions

can curtail weight loss, including underactive thyroid, depression, diabetes, and medications (including corticosteroids and the hormones in certain birth-control pills and postmenopausal hormone replacement therapy).

• Don't overestimate how much physical activity you're getting. Buy an inexpensive step counter or pedometer. Monitor your daily mileage and increase by five hundred steps.

• Problem-solve your way around the wall. Ask yourself the following questions, and write your answers in your notebook or computer file.

1. What is your biggest weight-loss problem right now? Make it specific. For example, I stick to my diet during the week but blow it on weekends.

2. List every way you can think of to solve this problem. The more solutions you list, the greater your chance of finding the one that will work best for you. For instance, to avoid weekend overeating, you might volunteer at a hospice or library or not do your grocery shopping until Monday so your cupboards remain bare over the weekend.

Read over your solution list and put a check by the solutions that make the most sense for your lifestyle. Pick one solution and implement it this week. If after a month this solution has failed you or you have failed it, read over your list again, and pick the next one on the list.

85

Counter Resistance

As you shed pounds, your body resists further losses. This physiological response, which may have once saved our ancestors from starving in times of famine, may trap you in a weight-loss rut. The best way out: counter resistance with resistance training. The more calorie-burning lean muscle tissue you have, the more calories you burn, even when resting. For each pound of muscle you gain, you'll burn thirty-five to fifty calories more a day—enough to reignite your metabolic engine so you keep losing weight.

The only way to build muscles is to demand more of them than you usually do. If you have not been working your muscles systematically, you should see a fairly rapid increase in strength within about six to eight weeks. If you're worried that working with weights will make you look heavier rather than leaner, fear not. Men bulk up when they pump iron because of the hormone testosterone and the larger number of muscle fibers in their muscles. As they tone their muscles, many women look leaner even without losing more weight.

You can strengthen and build muscles with free weights or resistance equipment at a gym. A research study that compared women working out at home with another group going to a gym found a definite home-turf advantage, with more of the at-home exercisers sticking with their shape-up program. On the other hand, gyms or health clubs offer more equipment and options so exercise is less tedious. We suggest you try both.

Wherever you work your muscles, vary the resistance (the amount of weight lifted), repetitions of each exercise, and sets (number of repetitions of the same movement or exercise). One day you might increase resistance and do fewer repetitions. On another you may go with lighter loads and do an additional set.

If you're still resisting resistance training, remind yourself that developing muscular strength and stamina lowers your risk of diabetes and heart disease, relieves back pain, strengthens joints and bones, boosts self-confidence, and enhances mood.

86

Constructive Living for Weight Loss and Maintenance

Constructive living, an educational approach to life developed by an American cultural anthropologist, David Reynolds, has its roots in Morita, a Buddhist-inspired therapy. Constructive living teaches that what you do today molds you for tomorrow. Focusing on negative feelings intensifies them, but doing something positive diminishes them. Whenever an unpleasant feeling comes into your consciousness, don't try to dismiss it, but rather think of a constructive action you might take.

To apply this approach to weight loss and maintenance, know what you want, do not act on negative feelings, and put your energy into constructive behavior (which may or may not be related directly to weight loss). For example, if you're feeling disgusted about weighing more than ever, it is not constructive to comfort yourself by eating. Instead, simply note your disgust with yourself, and then focus on a constructive action, such as a vigorous workout or paying bills. If you're upset because you can't fit into a favorite outfit, you might take constructive action by cleaning out your closet and giving clothes you no longer wear to a charity. Each time an uncomfortable feeling tugs at you, identify it, respect it, and take constructive action rather than acting on the feeling.

One of the lessons of constructive living is that what matters isn't what or how you feel, but what you do and accomplish. In several months, with the use of this approach, you will notice major changes in the way you eat—and in the way you live.

87

Five Ws and an H

If you do overeat or binge, resist the urge to beat yourself up and abandon all hope of ever losing weight. To regain some objectivity, think of yourself as a reporter, writing the "lede" or opening paragraph of a news story. Ask and answer the "five W's and an H": who, what, when, where, why, and how.

Think back to your fall off the weight-loss wagon and ask yourself:

Who? Did you eat alone or with others?
What? Exactly what did you eat? Estimate portions and servings.
When? Was this a snack, meal, midnight munch?
Where? In the kitchen, car, restaurant, at a bar?
Why? Tired, annoyed, anxious, happy, hungry, lonely?
How? Did you sit down and eat slowly? Or did you inhale your food as you rushed to do another chore?

The more information you have about your eating behavior, the more you'll be able to control it. Look at your answers and write in your notebook strategies for overcoming these pitfalls, such as restricting where you eat or measuring servings, to prevent lapses in the future.

88

Your Weight Karma

In the Buddhist and Hindu traditions, karma means that nothing happens by itself. Everything is a result of what has gone before. If unhealthy behavior and bad choices came before, what follows is an unpleasant event. If what came before is good and worthy, what follows is pleasant. Being true to yourself and making ethical choices determines your lot in the future.

When you reflect on the idea of karma in connection with your weight and lifestyle, think of what has gone before. Have you taken good care of your body? Have you kept it fit and fed it well? Or have you abused it with barrels of cookies and chips, vats of ice cream, mounds of cakes and pies? Have the choices and habits of the past created bad weight karma?

In addition to the karma of your past, there is the karma that will shape your future. Consider:

- Are you creating more pain and suffering for yourself by continuing to neglect your body or not working hard enough to repair the damage already done?
- Is the karma that your current lifestyle is creating the one that you want?

You *can* have a different life. As you begin or continue to make healthier choices, you will be creating good karma both for the present and future. Start the process, and enjoy a day, a week, a month, a lifetime of healthy living and good karma.

89
Boogie On

Do you want to build mental as well as physical muscles? Turn on the music during your workouts. According to new research from Ohio State University, listening to music while exercising helps to increase brainpower.

In the experiment, volunteers completed tests of both mood and verbal skills before and after two separate thirty-minute sessions on a treadmill—one in silence, one while listening to Vivaldi's *The Four Seasons*. After both sessions, the participants reported feeling better emotionally. However, the improvement in a test of verbal skill after listening to music was more than double than that following a music-less workout.

How can moving to music affect cognitive ability? Exercise in itself causes positive changes in the nervous system that may directly affect cognitive ability, say the researchers. Listening to music may do the same, but through different pathways, so the combination of movement and music provides much greater stimulation to the brain.

Next time you head for the walking path, treadmill, or gym, put on your earphones, turn on your radio or music player, and boogie on to benefit brain as well as body. If you don't have access to music, sing to yourself, or make up a chant like the ones military recruits grunt as they jog in formation. Try this one to keep yourself motivated as well as moving:

> *Look at me. I'm going strong.*
> *I can run the whole day long.*

90

Visualize Your Race

If you imagine a hypothetical event, such as winning an award or being selected to manage a project, you are more likely to consider it possible and make it happen. In studies of world-class athletes, those who practiced positive visualization performed better than those who exercised just as much but did not use this psychological technique.

However, it's important to visualize not just the final moment of triumph, but the actual steps and activities that lead up to it. Olympic gold-medal hurdler Edwin Moses used to visualize a complete 400-meter hurdle race, imagining himself crossing each hurdle and sprinting to the finish line. Sports psychologists believe that his visualization of the entire race was more effective than if he had just imagined the moment when the gold medal was slipped over his head. It motivated him to practice and helped him focus on performance rather than only victory.

Visualize yourself waking up full of confidence and determination and planning a day of healthy eating and exercise. See yourself eating slowly, enjoying each bite, and pushing back your plate when you first start to feel full. Visualize yourself sipping from a water bottle throughout the day. See yourself changing into workout clothes and moving gracefully through your Pilates exercises or jogging along your favorite path. Notice the sensations within your body and the sights and sounds around you.

Practice your positive visualization at least twice a day, once in the morning and once in the evening. The more detailed your vision of your positive behaviors, the more benefits you'll derive from the exercise. End each visualization with your personal equivalent of an Olympic gold medal—whether that's stepping on the scale with a smile, zipping yourself into a glamorous new outfit, or making a grand entrance at your next school or family reunion.

91

Social Psychology

Are parties your waistline's Waterloo? Do you wilt when a food pusher insists that you have a second helping? Can a waiter sweet-talk you into ordering three courses regardless of how hungry you are? If so, here are the fundamentals of a good defense:

• Do a dress rehearsal. The night before a big event, such as a holiday party or elegant dinner, rehearse the event in your mind. If you know Aunt Bea is bringing the world's best pound cake, plan how much you'll take—and what other dishes you won't sample. See yourself drinking water, putting your knife and fork on the table between bites, and saying no to an extra dollop of sour cream. Rehearse the moments most likely to lead to diet downfall, like the appearance of the dessert tray or the eggnog toasts. Come up with alternative scenarios, such as trying just one bite or sip, or spending more time on the dance floor and less near the buffet.

• When heading to a party, declare some foods off-limits. For example, decide that you'll eat pretzels but not chips, carrots but not cookies, shrimp but not pâté.

• Don't stand near the food.

• Pace yourself to eat more slowly than anyone else at the party or table.

• Watch what you're drinking as well as what you're eating. Alcohol not only adds extra calories but lowers inhibitions so you eat more. Alternate a glass of wine with a glass of mineral water or seltzer. (See chart on page 212.)

• Never talk with your mouth full, and find friends you enjoy talking with.

• Rehearse snappy comebacks. For example, "I can't eat another bite, but your food is absolutely delicious." Here are some effective responses you might rehearse and have ready:

• Is that all you're going to order?

　I'm trying to lose weight.

• Don't tell me you're dieting again.

　Just sticking with the program.

• This bread is wonderful. Have a small piece.

　No, thanks. I'm on a low-carb diet.

• You're no fun.

　I think I'm fun.

• How can you eat salad when we're eating pizza?

　Doctor's orders.

• Come on, everyone's ordering dessert.

　I'll have a bit of yours.

How Many Minutes to Work Off a Drink?

We're not saying don't drink. But be prepared to pay the price—in pounds or in sweat—if you have:

A glass of dry white wine (approximately 85 calories)

- Walk for 22 minutes (at 3 mph).
- Bicycle for 13 minutes (at 9.4 mph).
- Swim for 10 minutes (at 2 mph).

A martini (140 calories)

- Walk for 37 minutes.
- Bicycle for 22 minutes.
- Swim for 17 minutes.

A lite beer (105 calories)

- Walk for 28 minutes.
- Bicycle for 17 minutes.
- Swim for 13 minutes.

92
Log on to Lose Weight

Every month an estimated 5 million Americans log on to commercial web sites targeted to dieters. Why? Online dieting is convenient, anonymous, and available around the clock. It also draws on some of the same psychological principles we describe in *Think Thin, Be Thin*, including:

- **Monitoring food intake.** Many dieters use online calorie and carb calculators to record and evaluate what they're eating.
- **Posting a psychological journal.** Using e-names like dietgirl and skinnysue, dieters can express feelings that may be too emotionally charged to share with friends and family.
- **Tracking progress.** Some dieters post their weekly weights, down to the quarter pound, or before-and-after photos of the way (and weight) they were and how far they've come.
- **Finding support.** In various blogs and chat groups, dieters commiserate, exchange tales of setbacks and successes, and encourage each other to stay the course. Simply reading diet blogs can help you feel less lonely in your quest.

- **Information gathering.** Dozens of sites provide tips, programs, and research on every aspect of weight loss. Not all are reliable, but we list some of the authoritative and helpful sites in the Appendix.

If you want to turn your computer into a diet ally, look for more than fitness and diet suggestions online. In a study at Brown University, dieters who received weekly advice from behavioral therapists on the Internet lost three times as much weight as those who simply had access to information. The volunteers in this study followed a standard weight-loss regimen, including a diet of 1,200 to 1,500 calories per day and a minimum of 1,000 calories of exercise per week. Among those who received online support and advice from behavioral therapists, 45 percent—about twice the percentage of the education-only participants—lost at least 5 percent of their body weight. The reason may be that the extra support motivated them more than the information alone.

However, computers can't take the place of real-life support. In the Brown study, dieters lost an average of nine pounds in six months. By comparison, dieters lost an average of twenty pounds with one-on-one, face-to-face weight-loss counseling.

93
Aromatherapy: Take a Deep Whiff

People who lose their sense of smell and taste after head trauma typically gain ten to twenty pounds. Yet those who work in candy stores often say they aren't even tempted to eat chocolate. Why? Because odors affect your appetite. For example, you may feel especially full after eating a feast like Thanksgiving dinner not only because of the tasty foods that cross your lips but also because of the rich variety of scents that reach your nose.

According to neurologist Alan Hirsch, founder of the Smell and Taste Treatment and Research Foundation in Chicago, specific aromas can suppress rather than stimulate appetite and reduce cravings. In his studies, strong sweet scents such as chocolate often triggered feelings of hunger and led to overeating or binge eating, while "neutral" sweet smells actually curbed appetite. To test his theory, he asked 3,193 overweight people (mostly women) aged 18 to 64 to inhale a variety of "neutral" sweet smells, including banana, green apple, vanilla, and peppermint, three times in each nostril whenever they were hungry. They lost an average of five pounds a month. Similar research at the Human Neuro-Sensory Laboratory in Washington, D.C., also showed that inhaling certain scents can lead to weight loss.

How do scents affect weight? They may fool the brain into believing that you have eaten more than you did, so you feel full more quickly and eat less.

Although aromatherapy is still an experimental approach to weight loss, why not put it to the test? Try inhaling the odors of the foods you like best, preferably in a nonfood form, so you're not tempted to eat. Try fruit-scented candles or spicy potpourri. By filling your nose with the scent of delicious foods, you may be less likely to stuff your stomach with them.

94

Metabolism Management for the Long Haul

Do you complain about having a slow metabolism or having to fight your metabolism to lose weight? You have more control than you think.

Metabolism is the rate at which your body burns calories to sustain itself. Genetics does affect it; so do medical conditions such as thyroid disorders. Some people naturally have higher metabolisms and can eat more without gaining weight. If you aren't a naturally born rapid metabolizer, you still can speed up your own metabolism with a little effort. Here's how:

• Build more muscle tissue. Lean body mass turbocharges your metabolism so you burn more calories throughout the day. (See Tip 85.)

• Eat small meals and healthy snacks. Eating at regular times throughout the day actually burns off 10 percent more calories than skipping meals because eating itself increases metabolic rate. Many people do best eating five small meals rather than three "squares."

• Don't go too low if you're cutting back on fat. Extreme low-fat diets can affect hormone production and slow metabolism.

• Drink plenty of water. More than 70 percent of your body's functions require water; dehydration causes all your systems to slow down.

• Don't starve yourself. Without sufficient calories, your body cannibalizes muscle when it needs energy, and less muscle means a slower metabolism.

• Build miniworkouts into your day. If you sit at a desk or computer all day, take five minutes off every hour or two to walk down a few flights of stairs or do some wall push-ups or jumping jacks. (Note: These are supplements to, not substitutes for, your daily workout.)

95

Autopsy Diet Disasters

Maybe you tried low-carb last year, low-fat the year before, and a dozen diets du jour in the preceding decade. You may think of them as diet failures. We think of them as case studies that may help you succeed at long-term weight loss.

Look back on your diet experiences and "autopsy" what went wrong—and right. Start with the following questions, which you can answer in your notebook or computer file.

* What blindsided, distracted, demoralized, or otherwise derailed you on past diets?
* What excuses did you use when you went off previous diets?
* Who were the diet saboteurs who undermined your efforts?
* How did they sidetrack you?

Now focus on your current weight-loss program.

* What potential pitfalls do you anticipate? Have you encountered any so far?
* How did or will you overcome them?
* What are your backup plans in case something or someone unexpectedly tries to sabotage your current weight-loss program?

96
I've Got a Secret

We played this game in one of our weight-loss groups, and here's what we heard:
- "My secret is that I always get up around 2:00 a.m. and have cookies and milk."
- "I eat while I'm cooking a meal. By the time I'm ready to serve it, I'm already full. But that doesn't stop me from eating a complete dinner."
- "I drink a 64-ounce bottle of soda every day. I can't help myself."
- "I'll eat five or six marshmallows after lunch and dinner, even if I've had another dessert. Sometimes I'll have them with hot tea in the afternoon. I'm addicted."

What are your food secrets? Are they secretly sabotaging your weight-loss efforts? Are you willing to change any of them?

The woman in our group who snacked on cookies and milk during the night decided to drink a half glass of milk when she woke up hungry. The nibbling cook chews gum as she prepares dinner. The soda lover weaned herself from 64 to 32 to 16 to 8 ounces a day—and finally switched to chai tea.

Like most people, you probably have some food secrets. List a few. Think about them over the next few days.
Maybe you'll want to share them with a diet buddy or
weight-loss group. Maybe not. The important thing is
that you recognize and admit them to yourself. Decide if
the behavior is keeping you from your weight-loss goal.
You may want to change your secret.

97

Relapse Rx

A Brown University study followed a group of volunteers who had been exercising for at least twenty minutes three times a week. Two months later, 87 percent were still working out, but 13 percent were not. Psychological tests revealed one key difference between the two groups: The people who stopped exercising scored lower on measures of self-efficacy, the feelings of competence and control discussed in Tip 11. In addition, they listed fewer "pros" or advantages of exercising than those who stuck with the program.

One way to prevent—or recover from—relapse, the researchers concluded, is to reduce the number of "cons" so that people have less reason to drop out of an exercise program. If you've relapsed or feel you soon might, identify your cons and list ways to work over, around, or through them.

Here are some examples:

Cons	Countercons
Gym membership too expensive	• Check out a local Y or community center • Walk or jog outdoors • Invest in inexpensive hand weights
Self-conscious in exercise classes or gym	• Rent videos or DVDs so you can practice at home • Check out less intimidating environments, such as women-only gyms. • Invite a friend to work out with you.
Too busy	• Wake up half an hour earlier to get your workout done for the day. • Settle for half workouts if you can't do a full one. • Set aside exercise "appointments" on your schedule
Boring	• Mix it up. Walk one day; bike or jog the next. • Try something new, like tai chi.

98

The Gift

What happens when you lose weight? You feel great about yourself. You hold your body differently. Your stride changes. You convey to the world, "I like myself." And you do. You feel good and successful. When other challenges appear, you know you have the grit, stamina, and strength to deal with them. As you shape up and slim down, you give yourself a gift you may not have anticipated: resiliency.

When you get off the treadmill or finish your last lap in the pool, you may be a bit tired, but you have a renewed sense of self, a belief that you're strong and tough and can handle whatever comes your way. Just like your muscles, your resiliency has grown stronger.

Researchers who've studied trauma survivors have found that resilient people aren't necessarily braver or stronger than others, but they overcome their weaknesses and amplify their strengths.

Flex your resiliency muscle every day—pass up a fatty food, walk faster, and feed your mind as well as your body. Show that you can do more than merely survive: Thrive. Let that be the gift your weight loss gives you every day.

99

Six Ways to Keep Off Weight

Maybe you've reached your weight-loss goal. Maybe you're closer than ever. Sooner or later, you'll face a new problem: How do you keep the pounds you lost from coming back? These are our five favorite long-term strategies:

1. **Stay active.** In study after study, exercise has proven to be the key to lasting weight loss. Because exercise preserves muscle tissue, you'll continue to burn more calories all day every day. Keep setting new workout goals. Try new sports and activities. If illness or injury sidetrack you from jogging or weight lifting for a while, consult a trainer to find safe alternatives. Read entries that summarize what exercise can do. These will help motivate you to get back to an active life as soon as possible.

2. **Drink more.** Water is so essential to weight loss and maintenance that we think of it as "hydrotherapy." Water prevents bloating and fluid retention, creates a feeling of fullness, suppresses appetite, improves digestion, and helps the body metabolize stored fat. Some experts recommend drinking enough water every day to equal half of your body weight in ounces. If you weigh 160 pounds,

aim to drink 80 ounces a day. Drink fluids with each meal, and carry a water bottle with you at all times.

3. **Find new comfort foods.** Choose a variety of foods that are satisfying for you emotionally, but not high in calories. Good options include air-popped popcorn, vegetable soup, chocolate fruit sundaes (fresh fruit with a spoonful of rich syrup), hot chocolate (with skim milk), and Fudgesicles (creamy but low in calories). Rather than feeling deprived, you'll enjoy a sense of fullness some nutritionists describe as "abundant abstinence."

4. **Join a "tribe."** Surround yourself with people committed to a healthy, active, fulfilling life. Extend your horizons. Take a ceramics class or join a group of birdwatchers. Volunteer at a nursing home or library. Even if you're shy, exercise at a place and time where others are working out—a park on a Sunday afternoon or the gym on Wednesday evening.

5. **Reread *Think Thin, Be Thin*.** Because weight loss and maintenance is a lifelong project, continue to reinforce your diet or maintenance plan by reading various parts of this book again and trying more of the psychological techniques and strategies we describe. Make them a part of your life. Feel the power of meditation, visualization, self-hypnosis, journaling, positive self-talk, sensory representation, and daily affirmations.

6. **Look for joy and meaning beyond your food life.** Freud defined the essence of psychological well-being as the ability to love and to work. Tolstoy put it more poetically when he wrote, "One can live magnificently in this

world if one knows how to work and how to love, to work for the person one loves and to love one's work." Make love and work your priorities, and treat food as the fuel that allows you to do both.

100

Ten "Thinisms"

What's the word "thin" with the suffix "ism" attached? It's a word we invented to describe these inspirational phrases. Here are ten of our favorite thinisms. Copy the ones you like, and put them on index cards or Post-it notes on your refrigerator, your makeup mirror, your computer, or desk. Use them to keep yourself forever thin.

Wishing to have a better body is the first step to having a better body.

Weight is one of the few things people are happy to lose.

The more you practice restraint when eating, the more restraint you'll have.

Telling yourself you're destined to be fat destines you to be fat.

When people start losing weight, they go from being passive to passionate about their bodies.

Pretending that you aren't bothered by your weight doesn't make it any less bothersome.

Maybe you've become overweight so you'll have the pleasure of becoming thin.

With discipline comes freedom from weight.

Choose what you put in your mouth as carefully as you choose a pair of shoes.

Having too much weight is like having too much stuff. It gets in your way.

101

Honor Your Body

You've come a long way. You've learned to step back and observe yourself. You know how to change your thoughts and perceptions. You see the connection between what you think and how you feel and behave. Your relationship with food is different. You plan what you eat. You eat when you're hungry, not when you're upset or stressed. You've become more active. You feel more energetic and alive.

By reading *Think Thin, Be Thin,* you have changed the neuro-landscape of your brain. There is no going back. No longer can you rely on the same tired excuses for remaining heavy. No longer can you rationalize not working out. You know too much to settle for the way you were. This knowledge has become part of your brain and will keep you on track or gently nudge you back on track when needed.

By reading this book, by writing in your "Think Thin, Be Thin" notebook or computer file, and by completing the various assignments, you have learned to be respectful of your body and of yourself. In order to celebrate your new appreciation, plan a special day for yourself. You might choose to spend it hiking to a hilltop with a panoramic view or walking on a beach. You might prefer to pamper yourself with a facial or massage. Or you might give away all the oversized clothes you will never again wear.

From this day forth, vow to respect and take care of your wonderful body. And when you're tempted to eat beyond what is healthy and good for your body, remember these words: *Think Thin, Be Thin.*

Appendices

Determining Your Body Mass Index (BMI)

BMI	19	20	21	22	23	24	25	26	27	28	29	30	35	40
height (in.)							weight (lb.)							
58	91	96	100	105	110	115	119	124	129	134	138	143	167	191
59	94	99	104	109	114	119	124	128	133	138	143	148	173	198
60	97	102	107	112	118	123	128	133	138	143	148	153	179	204
61	100	106	111	116	122	127	132	137	143	148	153	158	185	211
62	104	109	115	120	126	131	136	142	147	153	158	164	191	218
63	107	113	118	124	130	135	141	146	152	158	163	169	197	225
64	110	116	122	128	134	140	145	151	157	163	169	174	204	232
65	114	120	126	132	138	144	150	156	162	168	174	180	210	240
66	118	124	130	136	142	148	155	161	167	173	179	186	216	247
67	121	127	134	140	146	153	159	166	172	178	185	191	223	255
68	125	131	138	144	151	158	164	171	177	184	190	197	230	262
69	128	135	142	149	155	162	169	176	182	189	196	203	236	270
70	132	139	146	153	160	167	174	181	188	195	202	207	243	278
71	136	143	150	157	165	172	179	186	193	200	208	215	250	286
72	140	147	154	162	169	177	184	191	199	206	213	221	258	294
73	144	151	159	166	174	182	189	197	204	212	219	227	265	302
74	148	155	163	171	179	186	194	202	210	218	225	233	272	311
75	152	160	168	176	184	192	200	208	216	224	232	240	279	319
76	156	164	172	180	189	197	205	213	221	230	238	246	287	328

Food Diary

Date	Time	Food or Drink	How Much	Place	With Whom	Feeling	Activity
10/3	8:00 A.M.	Oatmeal	1 cup	kitchen	alone	happy	watching TV

Notes

Introduction

Vastag, Brian. "Obesity is Now on Everyone's Plate," *Journal of the American Medical Association*, vol. 291, no. 10, p. 1186.

Tip 4

Christian, Kenneth W. *Your Own Worst Enemy* (New York: Regan Books, 2004.)

Tip 22

National Center for Health Statistics, www.nchs.gov.
"Global Strategy on Diet, Physical Activity and Health," World Health Organization http://who.int/dietphysicalactivity/publications/facts/obesity/en/
Working Group on Obesity. "Counting Calories." U.S. Food and Drug Administration. March 12, 2004. http://www.cfsan.fda.gov/~dms/owg-rpt.html#viii

Tip 25

Extensive research in recent years has documented the toll of obesity on health. Good summaries of the health risks of excess weight are available online. Among the most useful sites are:

NHLBI Obesity Education Initiative
www.nhlbi.nih.gov/about/oei/index.htm
American Obesity Association
www.obesity.org
American Dietetic Association
http://www.eatright.org.

Among the sources for the information on obesity, fitness, and health are the following recent studies: Manson, JoAnn. "A Fresh Look at Its High Toll," *Journal of the American Medical Association* 289, no. 2: 229, January 8, 2003.

Mokdad, A., et al. "Actual Causes of Death in the United States, 2000," *Journal of the American Medical Association* 291 (2004):1238.

Calle, Eugenia, et al. "Overweight, Obesity, and Mortality from Cancer in a Prospectively Studied Cohort of U.S. Adults," *New England Journal of Medicine* 348, no. 17 (April 24, 2003):1625.

Torpy, Janet. "Obesity," *Journal of the American Medical Association* 289, no. 14 (April 9, 2003):1880.

International Obesity Task Force (IOFT). "Controlling the global obesity epidemic," http://www.iotf.org.

Schwimmer, Jeffrey, et al. "Health-Related Quality of Life of Severely Obese Children and Adolescents," *Journal of the American Medical Association* 289, no. 14 (April 9, 2003):1813.

Peeters, Anna, et al. "Obesity in Adulthood and Its Consequences for Life Expectancy: A Life-Table Analysis," *Annals of Internal Medicine* 138, no. 1 (January 7, 2003):24.

International Obesity Task Force (IOFT). "Controlling the global obesity epidemic," http://www.iotf.org.

Tip 50

Hales, Dianne. *An Invitation to Health*, 11th ed. (Belmont, Calif.: Thomson/Wadsworth, 2004).

Tip 53

Pribram, Karl H. "The Neurophysiology of Remembering, *Scientific American* 220 (January 1969):73–86, 138. Paraphrased in Robert E. Ornstein, *The Psychology of Consciousness* (New York: Viking Press, 1972), 30.

Tip 54

Malkin, Amy, et al. "Women and Weight: Gendered Messages on Magazine Covers," *Sex Roles: A Journal of Research* 40, no. 7–8 (April 1999).

Tip 59

Fontaine, K. R., et al. "Years of Life Lost Due to Obesity," *Journal of the American Medical Association* 289, no. 2: 183, April 9, 2003.

Tip 70

Jakicic, John, et al. "Effect of Exercise Duration and Intensity on Weight Loss in Overweight, Sedentary Women," *Journal of the American Medical Association* 290: 1323.

Jakicic, J. M. "Exercise in the treatment of obesity," *Endocrinology and Metabolism Clinics of North America* 32, no. 4 (December 2003): 967.

Saris, W. H., et al. "How much physical activity is enough to prevent unhealthy weigh gain? Outcome of the IASO 1st Stock Conference and consensus statement," *Obesity Review* 4, no. 2 (May 2003):101.

Tip 71

McTigue, Kathleen, et al. "Screening and Interventions for Obesity in Adults: Summary of the Evidence for the U.S. Preventive Services Task Force," *Annals of Internal Medicine* 139 (2003):930.

Serdula, Mary, et al. "Weight Loss Counseling Revisited," *Journal of the American Medical Association* 289, no. 14 (April 9, 2003):1747.

Tip 75

Bray, George. "Low-Carbohydrate Diets and Realities of Weight Loss," *Journal of the American Medical Association* 289, no. 14 (April 9, 2003):1853.

Serdula, Mary, et al. "Weight Loss Counseling Revisited," *Journal of the American Medical Association* 289, no. 14 (April 9, 2003):1747.

Heshka, Stanley, et al. "Weight Loss with Self-help Compared with a Structured Commercial Program," *Journal of the American Medical Association* 289, no. 14 (April 9, 2003):1792.

Tate, Deborah, et al. "Effects of Internet Behavioral Counseling on Weight Loss in Adults at Risk for Type 2 Diabetes," *Journal of the American Medical Association* 289, no. 14 (April 9, 2003):1833.

Tip 78

Hu, Frank, et al. "Television Watching and Other Sedentary Behaviors in Relation to Risk of Obesity and Type 2 Diabetes Mellitus in Women," *Journal of American Medical Association* 289, no. 14 (April 9, 2003):1785.

Tip 80

Calle, Eugenia, et al. "Overweight, Obesity, and Mortality from Cancer in a Prospectively Studied Cohort of U.S. Adults," *New England Journal of Medicine* 348, no 17 (April 24, 2003):1625.

Tip 92

Tate, Deborah, et al. "Effects of Internet Behavioral Counseling on Weight Loss in Adults at Risk for Type 2 Diabetes," *Journal of the American Medical Association* 289, no. 14 (April 9, 2003):1833.

Tip 93

Hirsch, Alan. "'Sprinkle' Away Diet." Smell & Taste Treatment and Research Foundation, www.smellandtaste.org.

Tip 97

Sullum, Julie, et al. "Predictors of Exercise Relapse in a College Population," *Journal of American College Health* 48, no. 4 (January 2000):175.

Recommended Reading

Adler, Harry, and Heather, Beryl. *NLP* [neurolinguistic programming] *in 21 Days: A Complete Introduction and Training Program.* London: Piatkus, 1999.

Baldwin, Christina. *One to One: Self-Understanding Through Journal Writing.* London: Evans, 1992.

Beck, Judith S. *Cognitive Therapy: Basics and Beyond.* New York: Guilford Press, 1995.

Berne, Eric. *Games People Play.* New York: Random House, 1994.

Bloomfield, Harold H., and Robert K. Cooper. *The Power of 5.* Pennsylvania: Rodale Books, 1995.

Boorstein, Seymour, ed. *Transpersonal Psychotherapy.* 2d ed. Albany: State University of New York Press, 1996.

Burns, David D. *Feeling Good: The New Mood Therapy.* New York: Signet, 1980.

Burns, David D., Jr, and Paul D. Johnston, eds. *E-Prime III: A Third Anthology.* San Francisco: International Society of General Semantics, 1997.

Callahan, Roger. *Why Do I Eat When I'm Not Hungry?* New York: Doubleday, 1991.

Christian, Kenneth W. *Your Own Worst Enemy.* New York: HarperCollins, 2004.

Cialdini, Robert D. *Influence: Science & Practice.* 4th ed. New York: HarperCollins, 1998.

Corsini, Raymond J. *The Dictionary of Psychology.* Philadelphia: Taylor & Francis, 1998.

Deikman, Arthur J. *The Observing Self.* Boston: Beacon Press, 1982.

DeSalvo, Louise A. *Writing As a Way of Healing: How Telling Our Stories Transforms Our Lives.* Boston: Beacon Press, 2000.

Dodd, C H. *The Parables of the Kingdom.* New York: Charles Scribner's Sons, 1961.

Duyfe, Roberta. *American Dietetic Association Complete Food and Nutrition Guide.* New York: John Wiley & Sons, 2002.

Easwaran, Eknath. *The Mantram Handbook.* Tomales, Calif.: Nilgiri Press, 1998.

Ellis, Albert, and Robert Harper. *A New Guide to Rational Living.* North Hollywood, Calif.: Wilshire Books, 1975.

Fisher, Gerald H. "Measuring Ambiguity." *American Journal of Psychology* 80 (December 1967).

Fox, John. *Poetic Medicine: The Healing Art of Poem-Making.* New York: Tarcher Press, 1997.

Gilhooly, K.J. "Thinking." In *Encyclopedia of Human Biology,* ed. Renato Dulbecco. New York: Academic Press, 1991.

Glasser, William. *Choice Theory.* New York: HarperCollins, 1998.

Goldberg, Natalie, and Judith Guest. *Writing Down the Bones: Freeing the Writer Within.* Boston: Shambhala Press, 1986.

Goleman, Daniel. *Emotional Intelligence.* New York: Bantam Books, 1995.

Goleman, Tara Bennett. *Emotional Alchemy.* New York: Harmony Books, 2001.

Hales, Dianne. *An Invitation to Health.* 11th ed., Belmont, Calif.: Thomson-Wadsworth, 2004.

Hales, Dianne, and Robert Hales. *Caring for the Mind.* New York: Bantam Books, 1995.

Hales, Robert, and Stuart Yudofsky. *Textbook of Clinical Psychiatry.* 4th ed. Washington, D.C.: American Psychiatric Press, 2003.

Hanh, Thich Naht. *Living Buddha, Living Christ.* New York: Riverhead Books, 1995.

Helmering, Doris W. *Sense Ability: Expanding Your Sense of Awareness for a Twenty-First-Century Life.* New York: HarperCollins, 2000.

Hesley, John W., and Jan G. Hesley. *Rent Two Films and Let's Talk in the Morning.* New York: John Wiley & Sons, 1998.

James, Muriel, and contributors. *Techniques in Transactional Analysis for Psychotherapists and Counselors.* Reading, Mass.: Addison-Wesley, 1977.

Karpman, Stephen. "Fairy Tales and Script Drama Analysis," *Transactional Analysis Bulletin* (April 1969).

Keyes, Ken, Jr. *Handbook to Higher Consciousness.* 5th ed. Berkeley, Calif.: Living Love Center, 1975.

Kirschenbaum, Daniel S. *Weight Loss Through Persistence: Making Science Work for You.* Oakland, Calif.: New Harbinger, 1994.

Kornfield, Jack. *A Path with Heart: A Guide Through the Perils and Promises of Spiritual Life.* New York: Bantam Books, 1993.

Krech, Gregg. *Naikan: Gratitude, Grace, and the Japanese Art of Self-Reflection.* Berkeley, Calif.: Stone Bridge Press, 2002.

Lamont, Anne. *Bird by Bird: Some Instructions on Writing and Life.* New York: Random House, 1994.

Myers, David. *Psychology.* 7th ed. New York: Worth, 2004.

O'Connor, Joseph, and John Seymour. *Introducing Neuro-Linguistic Programming.* San Francisco: HarperCollins, 1993.

———. *Training With Neuro-Linguistic Programming.* San Francisco: HarperCollins, 1994.

Ornstein, Robert E. *The Psychology of Consciousness.* New York: Viking Press, 1972.

Paulhaus, L. Delroy. "Bypassing the Will: The Automatization of Affirmations." In *Handbook of Mental Control,* ed. Daniel W. Wegner and James W. Pennebaker. Englewood Cliffs, N.J.: Prentice-Hall, 1993.

Pennebaker, James W. *Opening Up: The Healing Power of Expressing Emotion.* New York: Guilford Press, 1997.

Persons, Jacqueline B. "Cognitive Behavior Therapy." In *Encyclopedia of Human Behavior,* ed. V. S. Ramachandran. New York: Academic Press, 1994.

Prochaska, James O., John C. Norcross, and Carlo C. DiClemente. *Changing for Good: The Revolutionary Program That Explains the Six Stages of Change and Teaches You How to Free Yourself from Bad Habits.* New York: William Morrow, 1994.

Rainer, Tristine. *The New Diary: How to Use a Journal for Self-Guidance and Expanded Creativity.* New York: Tarcher, 1979.

Reber, Arthur S., and Emily Reber. *The Penguin Dictionary of Psychology.* London: Penguin Books, 2001.

Reynolds, David K. *Constructive Living.* Honolulu: University of Hawaii Press, 1984.

———. *The Quiet Therapies: Japanese Pathways to Personal Growth.* Honolulu: University of Hawaii Press, 1980.

———. *Water Bears No Scars.* New York: William Morrow, 1987.

Stanley, Jason. *Killing the Food Monster.* Whitney, Tex.: The Food Monster, 2000.

Seligman, Martin E. *Authentic Happiness.* New York: Free Press, 2002.

———. *What You Can Change and What You Can't.* New York: Knopf, 1994.

Temes, Roberta. *The Complete Idiot's Guide to Hypnosis.* U.S.A.: Penguin Group, 2000.

Watzlawick, Paul, John Weakland, and Richard Fisch. *Change: Principles of Problem Formation and Problem Resolution.* New York: Norton, 1974.

Whitney, Eleanor, and Sharon Rolfes. *Understanding Nutrition.* 9th ed. Belmont, Calif.: Wadsworth-Thomson Learning, 2002.

Wholey, Dennis. *The Miracle of Change.* New York: Pocket Books, 1997.

Wilson, Paul. *Instant Calm: Over 100 Easy-to-Use Techniques for Relaxing the Body.* New York: Penguin Books, 1995.

Index

Authors' Note

Doris Wild Helmering is a psychotherapist who has been in private practice for thirty years. The author of nine books, she is a corporate speaker and executive coach, as well as a syndicated newspaper columnist, and on-air therapist. Ms. Helmering has appeared on *Oprah*, *Good Morning America*, and CNN. She lives in St. Louis, Missouri.

Dianne Hales is the author of thirteen trade books and the leading college health textbook, a contributing editor to *Parade*, and a freelance writer for a wide range of national magazines. She lives in the San Francisco Bay area.